Evidence-Based Group Work in Community Settings

There has been a strong recent trend towards incorporating evidence into Social Work practice in general, and into group work in particular. This trend has focused on the education of students in the use of evidence, development of evidence-based interventions, and discussion of how evidence can be used to improve practice. A limitation of most of this literature is that it has been written by researchers for the consumption of practitioners, limiting the ability of evidence-based practices to be incorporated into unique community settings and with specific populations. In spite of this difficulty, implementation of evidence-based practices continues quietly in practice settings.

This book describes efforts to integrate evidence into community settings, which have two foci. The first part details group models developed through collaborations between researchers and community agencies. Each chapter details efforts to implement, research, or review programs in community settings. The second part deals with issues around instruction and dissemination of evidence-based group work into practice settings. The volume makes a significant contribution to the discussion about evidence-based group work.

This book was published as a special issue of *Social Work with Groups*.

David E. Pollio, LCSW PhD, is the Hill Crest Foundation Endowed Chair. He has more than 25 years experience as a group work provider and researcher for adolescent and adult populations.

Mark J. Macgowan, LCSW, PhD, is with the School of Social Work at Florida International University in Miami and is Associate Director of the University's Community-Based Intervention Research Group. He has twenty-five years of group work practice and research experience, primarily with adolescents and with culturally-diverse populations.

Evidence-Based Group Work in Community Settings

Edited by David E. Pollio and Mark J. Macgowan

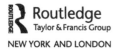
Routledge
Taylor & Francis Group

NEW YORK AND LONDON

First published in the USA and Canada 2011
by Routledge
711 Third Avenue, New York, NY 10017

Simultaneously published by Routledge
2 Park Square, Milton Park, Abingdon, Oxon, OX14 4RN

Routledge is an imprint of the Taylor & Francis Group, an informa business

This book is a reproduction of *Social Work with Groups*, vol. 33, issue 2/3. The Publisher requests to those authors who may be citing this book to state, also, the bibliographical details of the special issue on which the book was based.

Typeset in Garamond by Value Chain, India

British Library Cataloguing in Publication Data
A catalogue record for this book is available from the British Library

ISBN13: 978-0-7890-3851-7 (h/b)
ISBN13: 978-0-7890-3853-1 (p/b)

Contents

From the Editor

It is with pleasure that I introduce this edited collection, that is devoted to evidence-based group work practice. The editors David Pollio from The University of Alabama and Mark Macgowan from Florida International University have written and lectured extensively on social work practice, research and evidence-based group work. In joining together for this book, this "dynamic duo" has done a masterful of job of gathering, organizing and framing this illuminating work written by a diverse group of authors who are located in practice and educational settings all across the United States and in Canada and Korea.

In their introduction, Pollio and Macgowan assert that it is their mission to offer information and illustrations that will be of value to those working in "real-world settings." They have accomplished their goal.

Readers will be treated to a rich menu of practice settings, approaches and perspectives on evidence-based group work, presented by a learned group of practitioners, educators and researchers. This book is organized into two parts that present first, collaborations between researchers and those leading and working in community-based agencies; and second, educational ideas and approaches to best disseminate information about evidence-based group work in supervisory, classroom, administrative and agency-board-room-settings.

I am proud to present this lively, thought-provoking collection. It is my wish that this book will inspire others to write and submit manuscripts, to the journal, *Social Work with Groups*, that are dedicated to evidence-based practice in group work.

And so, without further adieu and with great anticipation, I welcome you to Pollio, Macgowan and Company's "Evidence-Based Group Work in Community Settings."

Andrew Malekoff
Editor-in-Chief

Introduction
to Evidence-Based Group Work in
Community Settings

Integrating evidence-based practice in social work in general, and in group work in particular, is an old and recent movement. Identifying client-level outcomes and examining the effectiveness of our practice models dates back to the beginning of professional social work. Nowhere has this been more evident than in group work. Robust clinical research on the effectiveness of specific group models has played a central role in social work research, so much so that a review of intervention trials found that more than half of the trials conducted by social work researchers were group based (Fortune & Reid, 1999). Well before the current movement in social work education toward evidence-based practice, there was a yearly meeting focused on empirical group work that met yearly for almost two decades.

In spite of the acceptance by the rest of the field of social work of the importance of developing evidence-based interventions and educating our future practitioners in incorporating evidence into practice, there have been roadblocks that have detracted from the dissemination of evidence-based practices into community settings. First, there is the now well-accepted problem that many of our best practices developed by researchers through traditional efficacy/effectiveness-focused approaches do not translate well into the "real world" of practice. This has led to the "translational research" movement, which emphasizes partnerships between researchers and practitioners in developing evidence-based treatments for the real world of practice. Again, this is not a new endeavor in group work; there are good examples of collaborative research-practice efforts in group work written well over 15 years ago (Galinsky, Turnbull, Meglin, & Wilner, 1993).

Second, although the need to educate practitioners in how to do evidence-based practice has led to several texts on how to teach evidence-based practice (including one by the co-editor, Macgowan, 2008), this has led to neither a clear pedagogy (or andragogy, as we argue subsequently) nor evidence that this approach is more effective than traditional approaches. In effect, we are touting a new paradigm—as Howard, McMillen, and Pollio (2003) did in the first Social Work publication on this topic—without submitting it to the same rigor that we urge in espousing evidence-based practices. We have not subjected the model to the test, in part because educationally it remains relatively ill defined. The Emperor simply does not have any clothes!

When the Editor-in-Chief Andrew Malekoff of *Social Work with Groups* approached us with the idea of guest editing this volume on evidence-based group work in community settings, we became very excited by the possibilities. Rather than continuing to contribute to the academic discussion, we could use the journal's focus on practice and its commitment to providing information that is useful in real-world settings to facilitate a discussion that might be useful and scientifically valid to community group workers and educators. We were also hoping to provide material that would help remove some of the material forming the two roadblocks detailed above. If the material would not be sufficient to remove the roadblocks completely, we were hoping that the discussions might help reduce them, or at least help us to go around them. If you allow us to stretch our metaphors, we were not trying to clothe the Emperor in ermine, but perhaps allow him some options in foundation garments.

This volume includes 10 articles that we think are scientifically interesting and useful to practitioners and to educators. We begin with a series of articles that detail group models developed through collaborations between researchers and community agencies. The first article by Marsiglia and colleagues presents their REAL groups for Latino children, a small-group intervention for at-risk children in their keepin' it REAL program. Next, Smith and Hall present a discussion of challenges to implementing their strength-oriented family therapy (SOFT) multifamily group model for adolescent substance users in a community setting. Mishna, Muskat and Wiener present a thorough review and discussion of the development and implementation of their school-based groups for students with learning disabilities, which includes preliminary evaluation data. Their discussion complements Smith and Hall's, as well as echoing many of the same themes. Next, Bidgood and colleagues present their Supporting Tempers, Emotions and Anger Management (STEAM) program for children conducted in a community agency setting. Finally, Duncan and Klinger present a review of evidence-based programs in group, school, and community settings for children with autism-spectrum disorders.

These articles share common features. Beyond a proclivity for catchy names, each details efforts to implement, research, or review programs in community settings. Although it was not our intention, these articles also focus on some level on issues involving children and/or adolescents. All include some attention to the challenges of conducting standardized (mostly manualized) interventions within their community–academic partnership. All articles pay attention to the various systems that affect the child's behaviors, such as families and schools, and on the context in which the issue of clinical plays out, such as in ethnic minority populations. Rather than controlling for these differences (as would be the case in efficacy/effectiveness-focused research) or translating the interventions into their settings, these articles either incorporate context within the model or spend considerable attention exploring the way context affects the interventions. We also believe that the groups or programs detailed in this first set of articles will be of interest to readers working with populations with these problems.

The second set of articles deal with issues around instruction and dissemination of evidence-based group work into practice settings. To begin, we include two pieces written by the co-editors focusing on instruction in evidence-based group work. The first details an integrated educational model on evidence-based group work. This model includes attention to how evidence-based group work principles integrate with skill development in the classroom, and how both can facilitate improved practice behavior. We deliberately choose the term *andragogy* over the more traditional *pedagogy* in that the model incorporates an adult-learner approach. We follow this presentation with an example of how the evidence-based practice model developed by Macgowan is incorporated in a master's level group-work practicum experience. Following this, we present two discussions of challenges around implementing evidence-based practice in community settings. This includes a second article by Muskat, Mishna, and colleagues that uses the experience detailed in their earlier article on developing their manualized group as a means to develop practice principles for enlisting agency staff in providing evidence-based group work. We also include an article by Krauss and Levin on a group-based intervention developed at Washington University in St. Louis to educate administrators on implementation of evidence-based practice.

We conclude with an article by Sheldon Rose and Hee-suk Chang on motivating clients in treatment groups. Using—as he has across his career— the best available evidence, Rose discusses this important issue in a practical, applied manner. We have included this article for two reasons. First, it provides recognition that despite the importance of manuals, "evidence" includes much beyond randomized clinical trials and quasi-experimental designs. Group work has had a long tradition of attending to issues around group dynamics, and this article reminds us that we need to attend to factors not often captured in standard scientific models. It echoes the writings on the importance of group work instruction beyond manualized practices.

Of equal importance, this article again reminds us that the evidence-based practice movement in social group work predates our current attention, and that the level of sophistication provided by the previous generations of empirical group work researchers in many ways remains of greater applicability than the current focus on manualized interventions. For pioneers such as Sheldon Rose, Charles Garvin, and Maeda Galinsky (to name only a few who have influenced the guest editors), the issues raised across the articles included here are very familiar to readers. We owe them a debt for beginning and sustaining the process of understanding how evidence-based practice is very much a central historical feature of group work. Although we think this volume makes a contribution to the discussion, the limitations and challenges outlined in each article remind us that there is much work to be done before we have a clear pathway to fully realized evidence-based group work in community settings.

David E. Pollio
Mark J. Macgowan
Editors

REFERENCES

Fortune, A. E., & Reid, W. J. (1999). *Research in social work* (3rd ed.). New York: Columbia University Press.

Galinsky, M. J., Turnbull, J. E., Meglin, D. E., & Wilner, M. E. (1993). Confronting the reality of collaborative practice research: Issues of practice, design, measurement, and team development. *Social Work, 38*(4), 440–449.

Howard, M. O., McMillan, C. J., & Pollio, D. E. (2003). Teaching evidence-based practice: Toward a new paradigm for social work education. *Research on Social Work Practice, 13*(2), 234–259.

Macgowan, M. J. (2008). *A guide to evidence-based group work.* New York: Oxford University Press.

Part I: Group Models Developed from Collaborations Between Researchers and Community Agencies

Real Groups: The Design and Immediate Effects of a Prevention Intervention for Latino Children

FLAVIO F. MARSIGLIA and VERÓNICA PEÑA

Arizona State University, Phoenix, Arizona, USA

TANYA NIERI

University of California, Riverside, California, USA

JULIE L. NAGOSHI

Arizona State University, Phoenix, Arizona, USA

This article describes the development and immediate effects of a small-group intervention designed to complement a school-based prevention program for children and youth. The REAL Groups intervention is the result of a partnership with predominately Mexican American schools located in the central city neighborhoods of a southwestern U.S. metropolitan area. The group members (N = 115) were fifth graders from six central city schools. Group members were identified and referred by their teachers as in need of additional support beyond the keepin'it REAL classroom-based substance abuse prevention intervention, or they were invited by the referred students. The REAL Groups followed a mutual aid approach, and Masters in Social Work student interns trained in the REAL Groups intervention served as the group facilitators. This article describes the small-group intervention and provides an initial report on the results by comparing the small-group members (n = 115) with Mexican-heritage classmates (n = 306) who only received the classroom-based keepin' it REAL prevention intervention. This is a feasibility study in preparation for the follow-up study with seventh graders. As expected due to the low drug-use rates reported by fifth-grade participants, the effectiveness results were inconclusive. The immediate findings, however,

*provide important information about the design and evaluation of
culturally specific group interventions with acculturating children.
The article provides important methodological and practice implications for small-group school-based interventions as well as
recommendations for future research.*

INTRODUCTION

The intervention described in this article evolved as part of ongoing efforts
to respond to unacceptably high substance-use rates among adolescents
(Johnston, O'Malley, Bachman, & Schulenberg, 2007). Recent research
shows that use rates among younger children are also increasing, and
their rates and prodrug attitudes are the precursor of future use (Donovan,
2007). These trends are found across all ethnic groups, but the drug abuse
literature tends to present Latino immigrant children across the age spectrum
as protected from substance use (de la Rosa, 2002; Warner et al., 2006).
Acculturation to mainstream American culture has been linked to prodrug
norms and attitudes of immigrant Latino children, leading to higher rates of
substance use (Kulis, Yabiku, Marsiglia, Nieri, & Crossman, 2007; Marsiglia &
Waller, 2002). On the other hand, greater identification with culture of
origin has been shown to be protective against substance use (Holley,
Kulis, Marsiglia, & Keith, 2006; Marsiglia, Kulis, Hecht, & Sills, 2004). The
dislocation produced by migration and the subsequent acculturation process
appear to play an important role in the alcohol and other drug-use trajectory
of adolescents, but less is known about the experience of younger children
and when is the best time to intervene.

Despite a growing recognition of the risk effects of acculturation and
the protective elements within cultures of origin, most prevention programs
do not clearly integrate culture in their interventions (Gosin, Marsiglia, &
Hecht, 2003). One notable exception is keepin' it REAL (Hecht et al., 2003;
Marsiglia et al., 2005), a culturally grounded school-based prevention program that is recognized by the U.S. Substance Abuse and Mental Health
Services Administration (SAMHSA) as a model program. Keepin' it REAL is
a 10-lesson intervention targeting preadolescents, implemented by trained
teachers, and accompanied by instructional videos, scripted and filmed by
youth. The program aims at preventing substance use by developing children's capacity to resist drug offers with the REAL (refuse, explain, avoid,
and leave) resistance strategies. The main premise of the intervention is that
many children initiate substance use not because they desire to use drugs

but, rather, because they lack the necessary social skills to successfully resist drug offers (Gosin et al., 2003).

As a universal prevention program (Substance Abuse and Mental Health Services Administration, 2003), keepin' it REAL takes place in regular classrooms within schools across the full spectrum of substance-use risk of the students. The program developers designed REAL Groups as a companion of the larger intervention to address the variation in risk among individual students and to target specifically children that appear to be more vulnerable to use drugs before entering adolescence. The research team, in partnership with the schools, designed and field tested the REAL Groups intervention guided by the following two exploratory hypotheses:

Hypothesis 1: Students in the REAL Groups will report greater cultural pride, higher self-esteem, and a stronger sense of mutual aid at the completion of the group sessions, relative to baseline. Even though they were at higher risk for substance use, by the time REAL Groups' members reach middle school they will be expected to report similar use rates of alcohol, tobacco, and other drugs than students who only received the classroom-based intervention.

Hypothesis 2: Students identified by their teachers as being at risk and who participate in the classroom-based and the companion small-group interventions will report similar substance use outcomes to those students who received only the classroom-based intervention.

THE MUTUAL AID APPROACH

The REAL Groups intervention follows a mutual aid approach to social work with groups. Mutual aid draws on resilience research, which highlights the value of social support networks and reciprocity in protecting children from negative outcomes and in facilitating their successful development (Bernard, 2004; Lee, 1986; Werner, 1989). Mutual aid is a mechanism for deriving effective support from the group members and for facilitating the creation of support networks (Shulman, 1984). Connections, relationships, and social networks provide the social capital needed to support children through their school adjustment process, and in the case of immigrant children through their acculturation process (Stanton-Salazar, 2001; Stanton-Salazar & Spina, 2003, 2005). In the mutual aid approach, group participants learn and receive support mostly from the other group members; the group facilitator's role is to support the emergence of the group process (Gitterman, 2005). A positive group process provides the stage for a fluid exchange of thoughts and experiences. Group members encourage and challenge each other through mutual aid, resulting in a collective approach to helping.

Mutual aid strengthens children's interpersonal relationship skills, further develops their personal identity, and prepares them for adolescence's decision-making situations (Bernard, 2004; Bogenschneider, 1996; Hair, Jager, & Garret, 2002; Malekoff, 2007). Mutual aid groups encourage children to connect with peers, express their personal power, and practice "equity and inclusion" (Bernard, 2004, p. 126). Mutual aid groups meet children's developmental needs and assist them to acquire critical-thinking skills, to strengthen their interpersonal relationship skills, and to develop a democratic orientation.

Mutual aid is the appropriate approach to apply with immigrant children coming from communities experiencing dislocation and stressful transitions (Steinberg, 2002). Participating in mutual aid groups enhances the ability of immigrant children to connect with peers going through similar processes (Marsiglia, 2002). Group members learn to identify shared values connected to their culture of origin; and at the same time, they can share with each other possible contradictions they experience between home, school, and peers' expectations. This approach allows group participants to contextualize risky situations by identifying challenges, protective factors, and in the case of the REAL Groups learn and rehearse specific drug resistance strategies within a cultural context.

The small-group component follows a culturally grounded orientation—that is, the lessons taught are rooted in the cultural values and norms of the community of origin (Marsiglia & Kulis, 2009). The children learn how to integrate and discuss norms and values of their culture of origin—in this case Mexican/Mexican American culture—as a resource or strength protecting them from drug use. In keeping with the developmental needs and assets of the target age group, the REAL Groups address peer relationships and interactions, prosocial behaviors, school and neighborhood adjustment, and group membership issues (Masten & Coatsworth, 1998; Phinney, Baumann, & Blanton, 2001; Phinney, Horenczyk, Liebkind, & Vedder, 2001; Phinney, Romero, Nava, & Huang, 2001).

REAL Groups: The Design and Implementation of the Small-Group Component

The REAL Groups intervention applies a variety of strategies to incorporate the mutual aid approach. Structured activities offer opportunities to generate relevant group thinking, whereas the group process facilitates reciprocity and authentic dialogue between the group members. Facilitators support group members' active participation through brainstorming, listening, evaluating options, planning, rehearsing, role-playing, applying information, and reflecting on life experiences and life choices (Gitterman, 2004; Hart, 1990). The group process promotes reciprocity by emphasizing the common needs of the members and by facilitating the development of multiple helping relationships as members give and receive support from their fellow group members.

The Role of the Group Facilitator

In the REAL Groups, group authority is decentralized and members support each other by sharing their skills and strengths (Steinberg, 1999). The facilitator engages group members as trustworthy experts on the acculturation process, school, and home experiences. The group facilitator supports members to make their voices heard and to exercise their power and potential within the safety of the group (Freire, 1998). Facilitators encourage ownership of the group by posing questions to engage students in the teaching–learning process, and by avoiding lecturing to allow students' active engagement in setting the direction of the group. Passivity, or the traditional classroom role of spectator, is consistently discouraged; instead, group members are encouraged to engage in transformative discourse and to question the master narrative's message that drug use is normative (Macedo & Freire, 2003).

The group facilitator makes members accountable for their participation. Active engagement supports the group members' ability to resist the negation of culture or origin and expands their prosocial behaviors (Freire, 1998). The dialogical method (i.e., discussion and critical thinking) teaches group members to rely on others when making decisions and allows students to connect their individual decision-making processes with their families, peers, and communities. For example, through discussion students in the small-group component learn that the belief that using drugs brings shame to the family might not be unique to their family, but instead the antidrug value may be common among most families.

REAL Groups participants received the standard teacher-taught classroom-based keepin' it REAL intervention and, in addition, took part in the 8-week psychosocial group, comprising approximately 10 children and meeting during school hours. The facilitators of the REAL Groups were masters-level social work graduate students who received intensive training in the manualized curriculum and the mutual aid approach to group work by the developers of the small-group intervention. A senior MSW group worker provided the facilitator with ongoing supervision.

Manual Content

The REAL Groups manual provides eight detailed group sessions and general instructions on how to engage participants in discussing their experiences related to the process of acculturation at their appropriate developmental level. The manual helps the facilitators connect the learned strategies with the participants' experiences and their daily lives (Fedele, 2004a, b; Masten & Coatsworth, 1998). The key topics in the eight sessions are

1. When you do not know – fostering mutuality in relationships
2. What is in a name? – recognizing and asserting personal needs linked to culture of origin
3. Let's make room for everyone – balancing uniqueness with inclusion
4. Where are you from? – valuing the self and the history of migration
5. My neighborhood – valuing the self as a resource to others
6. Dream and act – maintaining a vision of the future and acting to realize that vision
7. My family and friends – cultivating a sense of belonging
8. You can count on me – connecting with support networks.

The group sessions help students discuss, rehearse, and apply the REAL resistance strategies to real-life situations connected with aspects of their culture of origin that protect them from risk, such as culturally supported antidrug norms. Students learn together, support each other, author their stories, and rehearse options and choices consistent with cultural norms learned at home and in their communities (Arrington & Wilson, 2000). The REAL Groups intervention aims at making explicit deeply held cultural values and potential value conflicts (Bogenschneider, 1996; Castro & Alarcón, 2002; Greene & Lee, 2003; Hair et al., 2002; Masten & Coatsworth, 1998). The group sessions provide members with opportunities to discuss, address, clarify, and redefine misconceptions and stereotypes about them and their communities of origin. This article reports on the design of the group intervention and its immediate evaluation of effectiveness. A more in-depth follow-up assessment of the same children will follow as group members' progress into middle school and their alcohol, tobacco, and other drug-use rates become more serious.

METHOD

Data for this study came from the Drug Resistance Strategies Project, a longitudinal randomized control trial of keepin' it REAL involving 30 center-city public schools and funded by the National Institute on Drug Abuse. The initial phase of the study included every fifth-grade classroom in the participating schools. The team secured active parental consent and student assent (in accordance with university and school district Institutional Review Board policies) from approximately 82% of the eligible students. University-trained survey proctors administered a 1-hour, written questionnaire for the evaluation of the classroom-based universal prevention program. Similarly, proctors administered a 30-minute written questionnaire in the REAL Groups for the evaluation of the indicated small-group intervention. The pretests were administered in Fall 2004, and the posttests were administered in Spring 2005, after the classroom-based intervention and REAL Groups were implemented. Students had a choice to complete the surveys in either English or Spanish. Survey administrators informed students that the surveys were part of a research project, their participation was voluntary, and their answers to the questions were confidential. More than 96% of the students with parental consent completed the surveys.

Sample Design

The subsample analyzed here included 421 consented students who were in the six schools that implemented the REAL Groups in addition to the classroom-based program. The sample was gender balanced (50% female). Ninety-five percent were aged 10 or 11 years. The same percent of participants (95%) was from low-income families, as indicated by their participation in the federal free or reduced-price lunch program at school. The majority (61%) self-identified as Mexican American or Chicano, whereas 37% self-identified as Mexican, and 2% self-identified as Mexican and some other group. More than one half (54%) were native-born children of immigrants, 26% were foreign born, and 19% were native-born children of native parents.

Teachers completed a 10-item referral form, modeled after the Search Institute's (2010) list of developmental assets for middle childhood. Teachers referred students with a more diffused self-image, lower social skills, known or suspected substance use, and/or exposure to substance abuse through family members. The referred students were encouraged to invite other classmates as a means of preventing the onset of iatrogenic effects common in homogenous groups (Dodge, Dishion, & Landsford, 2007). If all group members share an identified need or risk, it is possible that they could reinforce the shared risk factor, and thus the participants' behavior will not change in the desired direction (Felps, Mitchell, & Byengton, 2006).

Of the 421 students in the subsample, 115 participated in the REAL Groups, forming 12 small groups (two in each randomly selected school); the rest of the students ($n = 360$) became the default comparison group. The demographics of the group members resembled those of the total sample, with one exception. REAL Groups participants comprised slightly more males (53%) than females. The noted slight gender unbalance is not surprising given that teachers referred students, among other things, based on their substance use risk, and boys tend to be at higher risk for substance use (Dakof, 2000). Analyses related to Hypothesis 1 included only group members ($n = 115$), whereas analyses related to Hypothesis 2 included

TABLE 1 Means and Standard Deviations of REAL Groups Outcomes ($N = 115$)

	Pretest M (SD)	Posttest M (SD)
Cultural pride		
There is more than one right way to see life.	4.15 (.89)	4.23 (.84)
Not everyone's opinion matters.[a]	3.02 (1.37)	2.98 (1.36)
Each culture (race, ethnicity, nationality) in the U.S. adds something valuable to society.	3.79 (.97)	3.83 (1.03)
Self-esteem		
I have a number of good qualities.	4.10 (.92)	4.02 (.91)
I don't have much to be proud of.[a]	3.58 (1.31)	3.63 (1.30)
I have a positive attitude toward myself.	3.86 (1.18)	3.66 (1.07)
Mutual aid		
When I am afraid, I can admit it to other people.	3.32 (1.35)	3.36 (1.24)
If someone mispronounced my name, I would tell them the right way to say it.	4.17 (1.07)	4.28 (.97)
I talk about my ideas with other people, even if I think they might not agree.	3.69 (1.17)	3.63 (.99)
I don't really listen when people talk because I already know what they're going to say.[a]	3.47 (1.32)	3.44 (1.28)
I make better decisions after I hear other people's ideas.	3.62 (1.20)	3.75 (1.14)
Some people are scared for no reason.[a]	2.80 (1.34)	2.79 (1.13)
I don't have to like somebody to understand how they feel.	3.37 (1.34)	3.35 (1.24)

Note. [a]Higher posttest means were desired except for these items.

all the students in the schools where REAL Groups were implemented ($N = 421$) divided into intervention and comparison groups.

REAL Groups Outcomes

Analyses related to Hypothesis 1 examined three sets of REAL Groups outcomes: (1) cultural pride, (2) self-esteem, and (3) mutual aid. All items had five response options: *strongly agree, agree, neither agree nor disagree, disagree,* and *strongly disagree.* Table 1 provides a detailed listing of the three sets of items.

Substance Use Outcomes

For Hypothesis 2, the analysis examined 13 substance use attitudes and behaviors as outcomes of the classroom-based intervention. Posttest assessments took place after the implementation of the classroom-based intervention; high values represented undesirable outcomes, that is, indicating higher levels of substance use or stronger prodrug attitudes.

The surveys assessed the frequency of students' substance use in the last 30 days and the self-reported amount consumed of each substance. Participants will complete the same questionnaire in subsequent waves of data collection. The items are developmentally appropriate for middle child-hood through preadolescence (Hecht et al., 2003; Kandel & Wu, 1995). Students indicated the frequency of recent substance use by responding to separate questions addressing the number of times they used alcohol, cigarettes, marijuana, and inhalants (from $1 = 0$ *times,* to $6 = 40$ *or more times*). Students indicated the amount consumed by reporting how many drinks of alcohol (from $1 = none$, to $7 = more than 30$), cigarettes (from $1 = none$, to $7 = more than 20$), and hits of marijuana they had consumed (from $1 = none$, to $7 = more than 40$). The analyses treat answers regarding each substance separately. A baseline measure of the substance use out-come, captured at the pretest, was included as a control variable in the regression analyses.

In addition to measures of actual substance use, we examined an array of drug-use attitudes that are precursors of substance use (Elek, Miller-Day, & Hecht, 2006): prodrug personal norms, drug offer vulnerability, intentions to use substances, positive substance use expectancies, prodrug parental injunctive norms, and prodrug friends' injunctive norms. The six scales had good to excellent internal consistency (Cronbach's alpha coefficients of 0.83 to 0.97). The mean of three personal prodrug norms captured the students' opinions on whether use of alcohol, cigarettes, and marijuana was "OK" for someone their age. Responses ranged from 1 (*definitely not OK*), to 4 (*definitely OK*).

The self-efficacy and drug offer vulnerability scale (Kasen, Vaughan, & Walter, 1992) used the mean of three items that captured students' confi-dence in their ability to refuse drug offers. Students indicated the extent to which they were sure they would say *no* to an offer of alcohol from a "fam-ily member," an offer of a cigarette from "a kid at school," and an offer of marijuana from a "close friend." Responses ranged from 1 (*very sure*), to 4 (*not at all sure*).

The average of three items captured substance use intentions by whether the students thought they would use alcohol, cigarettes, and mari-juana in the coming weekend if they had the chance. Reponses ranged from 1 (*definitely no*), to 4 (*definitely yes*).

An average of three items captured the respondents' perceived bene-fits of substance use (positive substance use expectancies). Items included "Drinking alcohol makes parties more fun," "Smoking cigarettes makes peo-ple less nervous," and "Smoking marijuana makes it easier to be part of a group." Responses ranged from 1 (*strongly disagree*), to 4 (*strongly agree*) (Hansen & Graham, 1991).

Two items measured injunctive norms, which entail expected negative reactions from significant others to the student's use of substances (Hansen, Johnson, Flay, Graham, & Sobel, 1988). The average of three items captured students' perceptions of how angry their parents would be if they found out that they had drunk alcohol, smoked cigarettes, or smoked marijuana.

Responses ranged from 1 (*very angry*), to 4 (*not at all angry*). An average of three items captured students' report of how their best friends would react (friends' injunctive norms) if they got drunk, smoked cigarettes, or smoked marijuana. Responses ranged from 1 (*very negatively*), to 3 (*no reaction*), to 5 (*very positively*).

Covariates

A dichotomous variable captured whether the student participated in the REAL Groups (1 = *yes*, 0 = *no*). Age in years was an ordinal measure with responses ranging from 1 (*7 years*), to 9 (*15 years or older*). Gender was dichotomous with 1 (female) and 0 (male). Participation in the school's federal free or reduced-price lunch program served as a measure of socioeconomic status: 0 (*no participation*), 1 (*free or reduced-price lunch*). Usual grades received in school, a common predictor of substance use (Wright & Pemberton, 2004), was captured by an ordinal variable with responses ranging from 1 (*mostly Fs*), to 9 (*mostly As*).

The analysis followed a three-step strategy. First, we conducted paired-samples *t* tests to assess pretest-to-posttest changes in the REAL Groups outcomes (cultural pride, self-esteem, and mutual aid) among the 115 participants who completed the pre- and post-REAL Groups evaluations. Second, we conducted independent samples *t* tests to assess for differences in means in the pretest substance use outcomes between participants in the classroom program and the REAL Groups and participants in the classroom program only. Third, we conducted linear regression analyses to assess whether participation in the classroom program and the REAL Groups predicted more or less increases in posttest substance use than participation in the classroom program only.

RESULTS

Table 2 shows the pretest and posttest means and standard deviations of the REAL Group proximate outcomes of cultural pride, self-esteem, and mutual aid. Differences were in the desired direction, but the paired-samples *t* tests yielded no statistically significant changes in means on these variables from pretest to posttest.

Before testing Hypothesis 2, we tested the assumption that REAL Groups participants were in fact at higher risk for substance use at baseline. Table 2 contains descriptive statistics of the substance use attitudes and behaviors of the REAL Groups participants and the classroom-program-only participants. There were no statistically significant differences between the two groups, indicating that the REAL Groups participants were not significantly different

TABLE 2 Pretest Means and Standard Deviations, Classroom-Only and REAL Groups Participants ($N = 421$)

	Participants in Classroom Program Only ($n = 306$)	Participants in Classroom Program and REAL Groups ($n = 115$)
Amount consumed in last 30 days		
Alcohol	1.15 (.51)	1.15 (.50)
Cigarettes	1.05 (.33)	1.04 (.24)
Marijuana	1.04 (.40)	1.03 (.37)
Frequency of consumption in last 30 days		
Alcohol	1.11 (.38)	1.15 (.54)
Cigarettes	1.02 (.15)	1.04 (.31)
Marijuana	1.02 (.24)	1.03 (.37)
Inhalants	1.05 (.27)	1.03 (.18)
Drug offer vulnerability	1.84 (1.24)	2.02 (1.29)
Positive drug expectancies	1.39 (.71)	1.35 (.54)
Parents' prodrug norms	1.31 (.78)	1.26 (.79)
Friends' prodrug norms	1.96 (1.41)	1.79 (1.36)
Personal prodrug norms	1.17 (.38)	1.19 (.38)
Intentions to use substances	1.20 (.46)	1.22 (.43)

from nonparticipants in their vulnerability levels. This lack of difference remained, even after we excluded invited (or nonreferred) REAL Groups participants.

The fact that there were no differences in risk between the two groups (i.e., nothing to be offset) renders void the expectation of similar posttest outcomes because of the students' participation in the REAL Groups. It is possible that the REAL Groups intervention would have a booster or extra dosage effect, yielding superior outcomes for participants who received the classroom program and the REAL Groups, relative to classroom-program-only participants. We ran regression analyses to test this alternate hypothesis, as well as our original Hypothesis 2.

Table 3 contains ordinary least squares regression results assessing the effect of REAL Groups participation on last-30-day substance use amount and frequency, when controlling for gender (female), the usual grades received in school, current age, school lunch program enrollment, and baseline substance use. We found that REAL Groups participation was not associated with any significant differences in outcomes related to alcohol, cigarette, or inhalant use. However, REAL Groups participation positively predicted greater increases in marijuana use at the posttest, compared to participants in the classroom program only.

An examination of the covariates models presented in Table 3 reveals that baseline substance use positively predicted—for most substances—posttest substance use. Better grades in school were associated with lower

TABLE 3 Unstandardized Linear Regression Estimates and Standard Errors, Predicting Posttest Substance Use (N = 407)

	Amount			Frequency			
	Alcohol	Cigarettes	Marijuana	Alcohol	Cigarettes	Marijuana	Inhalants
REAL Groups participation	−.019 (.077)	.021 (.038)	.074* (.037)	−.013 (.069)	.032 (.036)	.097* (.043)	−.037 (.064)
Female	−.042 (.070)	−.026 (.035)	.003 (.034)	.042 (.062)	−.037 (.033)	.037 (.039)	.095 (.058)
Usual grades	−.012 (.020)	−.017+ (.010)	−.013 (.010)	−.017 (.018)	−.021* (.009)	−.013 (.011)	−.020 (.017)
Age	.141* (.062)	.038 (.031)	.048 (.030)	.082 (.055)	.040 (.029)	.109** (.034)	.099+ (.051)
School lunch participation	.021 (.065)	−.018 (.032)	−.012 (.031)	−.047 (.059)	−.020 (.031)	−.032 (.036)	−.061 (.054)
Pretest substance use	.298*** (.070)	−.034 (.055)	.161*** (.043)	.186* (.072)	.091 (.077)	.313*** (.066)	.243* (.113)
Intercept	.365*** (.320)	1.069*** (.165)	.755*** (.153)	.782*** (.286)	.963*** (.168)	.347+ (.180)	.621* (.287)
Adj. r^2	.047	.002	.050	.015	.016	.089	.019
N	401	401	407	401	404	406	407

+p < .10, *p < .05, **p < .01, ***p < .001

posttest substance use, but the effect was only statistically significant in the case of the frequency of cigarette use. Older students were associated with a greater amount of alcohol use and a greater frequency of marijuana use at posttest.

Another set of regression models examined the effect of participation in the REAL Groups on six substance use attitudes: drug offer vulnerability, use intentions, parents' prodrug norms, friends' prodrug norms, personal prodrug norms, and positive drug expectancies (results not shown in tables). Participating in the REAL Groups did not yield statistically significant effects for these outcomes. These results do not support the alternate hypothesis that the REAL Groups had a booster effect, improving outcomes for youth who received the REAL Groups and the classroom program.

DISCUSSION

This article describes the design and reports on the immediate evaluation of a small-group component created to supplement a school-based prevention program. The REAL Groups intervention provides additional support (extra dosage) to fifth-grade students perceived to be at higher risk for substance use and to increase their responsiveness to the classroom-based prevention program. Although program results were mixed and inconclusive, the current study is instructive in highlighting methodological challenges associated with the implementation and evaluation of a small-group intervention as a companion to a classroom-based intervention.

One key challenge encountered by the current study was that the referral procedures did not yield a high-risk participant group as intended. It is possible that the concepts of high-risk and substance use vulnerability do not apply to this very young age group with a high representation of low-acculturated Latino children. Some teachers may have referred students with discipline problems, rather than those at risk for substance use. However, were this the case, we might have seen baseline differences between REAL Groups participants and the sample at large, because discipline problems are commonly associated with higher substance use or prodrug attitudes (Drapela, 2005; Wright & Pemberton, 2004). It appears to be very difficult for teachers to identify higher risk fifth-grade students. It is possible that the items on the referral form, which were intended to help teachers identify the risk level of the students, were developmentally not well adapted, or may not have matched well the social setting or the cultural background of the participants.

The pattern of effects for many of the outcomes was in the desired direction, but the evaluation of the behaviors specifically targeted by the REAL Groups interventions (cultural pride, self-esteem, and mutual aid) did not yield conclusive evidence of significant behavioral change. The posttest was administered immediately after the small-group intervention, and the lack of follow-up measures later in time prevents us from assessing the REAL Groups' longer term impact. The small sample size of 115 cases with complete data undermined the power of the statistical tests used to identify significant differences. It is also possible that the outcome measures lacked the sensitivity to capture the small-group component's effects. On the other hand, the REAL Groups participants could have been in an ideal situation to benefit fully from a primary prevention intervention. The effects of the small-group intervention will be captured long term when risk behaviors intensify in middle school and high school due to developmental and contextual factors.

REAL Groups participants did not differ from their classroom-program-only peers in their alcohol, cigarette, and inhalant use rates and prodrug attitudes. We cannot conclude that the small-group component compensated for differential substance use risk, because we did not find baseline differences between the two groups. The increase in self-reported marijuana use among a small number of REAL Groups participants was unexpected. The between-groups differences may be due to chance; but alternatively, it may be an unintended iatrogenic effect of the REAL Groups. The teacher referral process may have somehow caused REAL Groups participants to feel singled out and to engage in behaviors they felt were expected from them—that is, to be referred to the group became a self-fulfilling prophecy. Additional data on students' perceptions of their participation in the groups could be useful in testing this hypothesis. Because the invited group members were very similar to the referred members in all key outcomes, there is a possibility that the inclusion of invited friends by the referred students may have had the unintended effect of augmenting the iatrogenic effect.

Children that are more vulnerable to use drugs tend to move faster through the drug-use continuum in comparison to lower risk groups. Thus, the group intervention might have had an effect in slowing down the small-group participants' progression into drug use, though we do note the surprising increase of marijuana use for some of them. Perhaps the indicated intervention should have focused on a smaller number of students with the greatest need in each classroom; by engaging so many students, the intervention may have not achieved its intended population.

When students in the experimental and comparison groups reach the seventh grade, the longer term prevention effects of the small-group intervention will be assessed more clearly. In the meantime, this article provides a detailed description of the approach and the possible methodological challenges practitioners and researchers might face while assessing the effects of a companion small-group intervention with acculturating children and youth.

Recommendations for Future Practice Research

Project teams need to conduct an in-depth examination of the measures and need to work very closely with teachers to explain the referral criteria and their rationale. Once teachers make referrals, research team members should review and discuss the referral list with teachers to ensure that the referred students meet the membership criteria for the intervention. Conducting a separate analysis of the referral forms could be useful in investigating and documenting an early detection of a lack of distinction between groups and in implementing a corrective action.

Practitioners should consider alternative research designs when researching the benefits of mutual aid groups. For an indicated prevention intervention, it is important to collect evidence that the targeted group is at higher risk for adverse outcomes than the nontargeted group. An alternative design could include using the pretest data to distinguish who was at a higher risk for drug use. It might also be beneficial to assign half the at-risk group to receive the indicated intervention and to continue with the classroom-only (universal) intervention with the other half, creating a more identifiable control group.

The psychometrics and cultural relevancy of small-group interventions need to be further developed, and it could be beneficial to include additional measures to capture participants' feedback and to document the group process more in-depth. Some of the questions in need of further exploration are: (1) Did participants feel part of the group? (2) Did they receive the aid of others? (3) Did they provide aid to others? (4) If so, how was that experience? (5) To what extent was the group transformative for the participants? Measures of students' personal perceptions of the experience might help to better capture its effects. It would also be helpful to integrate into the model the fidelity data collected through interviews and observations of the facilitators. Additional data about the facilitators such as gender, ethnicity, language abilities, and cultural competency will allow for a closer examination of the social worker's role.

Additional questions researchers/practitioners need to ask themselves are: (1) How does one select an at-risk group without creating stigma? (2) Are the resources available for implementing the intervention? (3) What are the benefits relative to the costs? (4) What elements of the intervention are particularly important for producing positive change? (5) Which elements should one strengthen? (6) How generalizable is the intervention?

The examination of the seventh-grader results—a developmental period characterized by spikes in substance use onset (Hornick, 2003)—will allow for a more comprehensive assessment of developmental differences and may offer findings that are more conclusive. Seventh graders will also allow the research team to better test the extra-dosage hypothesis.

The current study provided a snapshot of the design and performance of a small-group component based on the mutual aid approach and designed to supplement the primary prevention program keepin' it REAL. Given the implementation issues associated with referral of group participants, our assessment of the REAL Groups' effectiveness was inconclusive. Further research will assess how this innovative intervention addresses the needs of higher risk students who participate in the school-based universal prevention program. The current study also documents the complexities that arise when designing and evaluating interventions with younger children prior to significant engagement in measurable antisocial behaviors. Conducting prevention with younger children in small groups is necessary even when the effectiveness of such programs is not easily assessed through conventional methods. The challenges identified by the current study call for innovation and more tailored research models.

ACKNOWLEDGMENTS

The National Institute on Drug Abuse (R01 DA05629) supported this study, and the manuscript was developed at the Southwest Interdisciplinary Research Center with support from the National Center on Minority Health and Health Disparities (award P20 MD002316–01, F. Marsiglia, P. I.). The content is solely the responsibility of the authors and does not necessarily represent the official views of the National Institute on Drug Abuse, the National Center on Minority Health and Health Disparities, or the National Institutes of Health.

REFERENCES

Arrington, E. G., & Wilson, M. N. (2000). A re-examination of risk and resilience during adolescence: Incorporating culture and diversity. *Journal of Child and Family Studies, 9*(2), 221–230.

Bernard, M. E. (2004). Emotional resilience in children: Implications for rational emotive education. *Journal of Cognitive and Behavioral Psychotherapies, 4*(1), 39–52.

Bogenschneider, K. (1996). An ecological risk/protective theory for building prevention programs, policies, and community capacity to support youth. *Family Relations, 45*(2), 127–138.

Castro, F. G., & Alarcón, E. H. (2002). Integrating cultural variables into drug abuse prevention and treatment with racial/ethnic minorities. *Journal of Drug Issues, 32*(3), 783–810.

Dakof, G. A. (2000). Understanding gender differences in adolescent drug abuse: Issues of comorbidity and family functioning. *Journal of Psychoactive Drugs, 32*(1), 25–32.

de la Rosa, M. (2002). Acculturation and Latino adolescents' substance use: A research agenda for the future. *Substance Use and Misuse, 37*(4), 429–456.

Dodge, K. A., Dishion T. J., & Lansford, J. E. (2007). *Deviant peer influence in programs for youth: Problems and solutions.* New York: Guilford.

Donovan, J. E. (2007). Really underage drinkers: The epidemiology of children's alcohol use in the United States. *Prevention Science, 8*(3), 192–205.

Drapela, L. A. (2005). Does dropping out of high school cause deviant behavior? An analysis of the National Education Longitudinal Study. *Deviant Behavior, 26*(1), 47–62.

Elek, E., Miller-Day, M., & Hecht, M. L. (2006). Influences of personal, injunctive and descriptive norms on early adolescent substance use. *Journal of Drug Issues, 36*(1), 147–171.

Fedele, N. (2004a). Relational movement in group psychotherapy. In M. Walker & W. B. Rosen (Eds.), *How connections heal?* (pp. 174–192). New York: Guilford Press.

Fedele, N. M. (2004b). *Relationships in groups: Connection, resonance, and paradox.* New York: Guilford Press.

Felps, W., Mitchell, T. R., & Byengton, E. (2006). How, when, and why bad apples spoil the barrel: Negative group members and dysfunctional groups. *Research in Organizational Behavior, 27,* 175–222.

Freire, P. (1998). *Pedagogy of freedom: Ethics, democracy, and civic courage.* New York: Rowman & Littlefield Publishers.

Gitterman, A. (2004). The mutual aid model. In C. Garvin, L. Gutierrez, & M. Galinsky (Eds.), *Handbook of social work with groups* (pp. 93–110). New York: Guilford Press.

Gitterman, A. (2005). Building mutual support groups. *Social Work with Groups, 28* (3/4), 91–106.

Gosin, M., Marsiglia, F. F., & Hecht, M. L. (2003). keepin' it REAL: A drug resistance curriculum tailored to the strengths and needs of preadolescents of the Southwest. *Journal of Drug Education, 33*(2), 119–142.

Greene, G. J., & Lee, M. Y. (2003). A teaching framework for transformative multicultural social work education. *Journal of Ethnic & Cultural Diversity in Social Work, 12*(3), 1–28.

Hair, E. C., Jager, J., & Garrett, S. B. (2002). *Helping teens develop healthy social skills and relationships: What the research shows about navigating adolescents.* Washington, DC: Child Trends.

Hansen, W. B., & Graham, J. W. (1991). Prevention of alcohol, marijuana, and cigarette use among adolescents: Peer pressure resistance training versus establishing conservative norms. *Preventive Medicine, 20,* 414–430.

Hansen, W. B., Johnson, C. A., Flay, B. R., Graham, J. W., & Sobel, J. L. (1988). Affective and social influences approaches to the prevention of multiple substance abuse among seventh grade students: Results from Project SMART. *Preventive Medicine, 17,* 135–154.

Hart, M. U. (1990). Liberation through consciousness raising. In J. Mezirow (Ed.), *Fostering critical reflection in adulthood: A guide to transformative and emancipatory learning* (pp. 47–73). San Francisco: Jossey-Bass.

Hecht, M. L., Marsiglia, F. F., Elek, E., Kulis, S., Miller-Day, M., Dustman, P., et al. (2003). Culturally grounded substance use prevention: An evaluation of the keepin' it REAL curriculum. *Prevention Science, 4*(4), 233–248.

Holley, L., Kulis, S., Marsiglia, F. F., & Keith, V. (2006). Ethnicity versus ethnic identity: What predicts substance use norms and behaviors? *Journal of Social Work Practice in the Addictions, 6*(3), 53–79.

Hornick, R. (2003). Alcohol, tobacco, and marijuana use among youth: Same-time and lagged and simultaneous-change associations in a nationally representative sample of 9- to 18-year-olds. In D. Romer (Ed.), *Reducing adolescent risk: Toward an integrated approach* (pp. 335–343). Thousand Oaks, CA: Sage.

Johnston, L. D., O'Malley, P. M., Bachman, J. G., & Schulenberg, J. E. (2007). *Monitoring the future national survey results on drug use, 1975–2006. Volume I: Secondary school students* (NIH Publication No. 07–6205). Bethesda, MD: National Institute on Drug Abuse.

Kandel, D. B., & Wu, P. (1995). The contribution of mothers and fathers to the inter-generational transmission of cigarette smoking in adolescence. *Journal of Research on Adolescence, 5*, 225–252.

Kasen, S., Vaughan, R. D., & Walter, H. J. (1992). Self-efficacy for AIDS preventive behaviors among 10th grade students. *Health Education Quarterly, 9*, 187–202.

Kulis, S., Marsiglia, F. F., Elek, E., Dustman, P., Wagstaff, D., Hecht, M. L. (2005). Mexican/Mexican American adolescents and *keepin'it REAL*: An evidence-based substance abuse prevention program. *Children & Schools, 27*(3), 133–145.

Kulis, S., Yabiku, S. T., Marsiglia, F. F., Nieri, T., & Crossman, A. (2007). Differences by gender, ethnicity, and acculturation in the efficacy of the keepin' it REAL model prevention program. *Journal of Drug Education, 37*(2), 123–144.

Lee, J. A. B. (1986). Seeing it whole: Social work with groups within an integrative perspective. *Social Work with Groups, 8*(4), 39–50.

Macedo, D., & Freire, P. (2003). Rethinking literacy: A dialogue. In A. Dardar, R. Torres, & M. Baltodano (Eds.), *The critical pedagogy reader* (pp. 354–365). New York: Routledge.

Malekoff, A. (2007). *Group work with adolescents: Principles and practice* (2nd ed.). New York: Guilford Press.

Marsiglia, F. F. (2002). Navigating in groups . . . experiencing the cultural as political. *Social Work with Groups, 25*(1/2), 129–137.

Marsiglia, F. F., & Kulis, S. (2009). *Diversity, oppression, and change: Culturally grounded social work.* Chicago: Lyceum Books.

Marsiglia, F. F., Kulis, S., Hecht, M. L., & Sills, S. (2004). Ethnicity and ethnic identity as predictors of drug norms and drug use among pre-adolescents in the Southwest. *Substance Use and Misuse, 39*(7), 1061–1094.

Marsiglia, F. F., Kulis, S., Wagstaff, D. A., Dran, D., & Elek, E. (2005). Acculturation status and substance use prevention with Mexican and Mexican-American youth. *Journal of Social Work Practice in the Addictions, 5*(1/2), 85–111.

Marsiglia, F. F., & Waller, M. (2002). Language preference and drug use among Southwestern Mexican American middle school students. *Children & Schools, 25*(3), 145–158.

Masten, A. S., & Coatsworth, J. D. (1998). The development of competence in favorable and unfavorable environments: Lessons from research on successful children. *American Psychologist, 53*(2), 205–220.

Phinney, J. S., Baumann, K., & Blanton, S. (2001). Life goals and attributions for expected outcomes among adolescents from five ethnic groups. *Hispanic Journal of Behavioral Sciences, 23*(4), 363–377.

Phinney, J. S., Horenczyk, G., Liebkind, K., & Vedder, P. (2001). Ethnic identity, immigration, and well-being: An interactional perspective. *Journal of Social Issues, 57*(3), 493–510.

Phinney, J. S., Romero, I., Nava, M., & Huang, D. (2001). The role of language, parents, and peers in ethnic identity among adolescents in immigrant families. *Journal of Youth and Adolescence, 30*(2), 135–153.

Search Institute. (2010). Retrieved March 3, 2010, from http://www.search-institute.org/system/files/40Assets_MC_O.pdf

Shulman, L. (1984). *The skills of helping individuals and groups* (2nd ed.) Itasca, IL: F.E. Peacock.

Stanton-Salazar, R. D. (2001). *Manufacturing hope and despair: The school and kin support networks of U.S.-Mexican youth*. New York: Teachers College Press.

Stanton-Salazar, R. D., & Spina, S. U. (2003). Informal mentors and role models in the lives of urban Mexican-origin adolescents. *Anthropology & Education Quarterly, 34*(3), 231–254.

Stanton-Salazar, R. D., & Spina, S. U. (2005). Adolescent peer networks as a context for social and emotional support. *Youth & Society, 36*(4), 379–417.

Steinberg, D. (1999). The impact of time and place on mutual-aid: Practice with short-term groups. *Social Work with Groups*, 22, (2/3), 101–118.

Steinberg, D. (2002). The magic of mutual aid. *Social Work with Groups, 25*(2), 31–38.

Substance Abuse and Mental Health Services Administration. (2003). *Science-based prevention programs and principles, 2002*. Rockville, MD: U.S. Department of Health and Human Services.

Warner, L. A., Valdez, A., Vega, W. A., de la Rosa, M., Turner, R. J., & Canino, G. (2006). Hispanic drug use in an evolving cultural context: An agenda for research. *Drug and Alcohol Dependence, 84S*, S8–S16.

Werner, E. E. (1989). High-risk children in young adulthood: A longitudinal study from birth to 32 years. *American Journal of Orthopsychiatry, 59*(1), 72–81.

Wright, D., & Pemberton, M. (2004). *Risk and protective factors for adolescent drug use: Findings from the 1999 National Household Survey on Drug Abuse*. Rockville, MD: Department of Health and Human Services, Substance Abuse and Mental Health Services Administration, Office of Applied Studies.

Implementing Evidence-Based Multiple-Family Groups with Adolescent Substance Abusers

DOUGLAS C. SMITH

University of Illinois at Urbana-Champaign, Urbana, Illinois, USA

JAMES A. HALL

University of Alabama, Tuscaloosa, Alabama, USA

Agencies that provide adolescent drug treatment services have reported increased demand to treat multiple families in groups. However, little attention has been paid to the challenges associated with implementing multiple-family group interventions for adolescent substance abusers. To address this gap in the literature, the authors discuss the implementation of multiple-family groups embedded within a promising multimodal intervention called Strengths-Oriented Family Therapy (SOFT). We provide a brief description of the system of care within which the SOFT multiple-family groups were developed and outline the process of implementation. The authors discuss challenges they faced implementing multiple-family groups in their partnership with a not–for-profit agency using Gotham's (2006) conceptual framework for the transfer of evidence-based models into community practice. The challenges included meeting state licensure standards, providing services in rural areas, supervising the multiple-family groups, and addressing therapist's concerns and assumptions about the model. The authors conclude with practical recommendations for others that are developing or implementing multifamily groups as adolescent substance abuse treatment models.

INTRODUCTION

Social workers have a long history of addressing client problems using an ecological approach. In the ecology for adolescents, the family system is recognized as a proximal influence on whether they abuse substances (Bronfenbrenner, 1986; Liddle, 2004; Steinberg, Lamborn, Darling, Mounts, & Dornbusch, 1994). Multimodal treatments that address family systems are gaining in popularity and are generally effective for treating adolescent substance abusers (Austin, Macgowan, & Wagner, 2005; Dennis et al., 2004; Liddle et al., 2001). Because of these robust findings, federal agencies that fund services are often requiring social workers to include family members in adolescent substance abuse treatments. Successful implementation of family-based interventions in typical practice settings, however, is a complex task and is best accomplished by a high level of collaboration between community practitioners and clinical scientists (Gotham, 2006; Liddle et al., 2006). In this article, we review one such collaboration between practitioners and researchers who implemented multiple-family groups (MFGs) as part of a promising multimodal intervention called Strengths Oriented Family Therapy (SOFT). We review the issues we encountered implementing multiple-family groups and argue that this neglected treatment modality is a viable way of including parents into adolescent substance abuse treatments.

MULTIPLE-FAMILY GROUPS

Definition

We define *multiple-family groups* (MFGs) here as groups where (1) multiple families attend groups together, (2) family-to-family peer support is encouraged, and (3) psychoeducation is not the sole focus. MFGs have been used by social workers with diverse populations including families of persons with schizophrenia, alcoholic couples, prisoners, and families in the child welfare system (Dennison, 1999; Meezan & O'Keefe, 1998). *Families* have been inclusively defined to account for all types of diverse family configurations. In this article, however, we discuss the implementation of MFGs that included adolescents aged 12 to 18 and their parents or guardians.

MFGs in Adolescent Substance Abuse Treatment

Although social workers have historically used MFGs with many different populations, few existing family-based treatments for adolescent substance abusers include MFGs as defined here (Dennis et al., 2004; Dennison, 1999; Hamilton, Brantley, Tims, Angelovich, & McDougall, 2001; Joanning, Quinn, Thomas, & Mullen, 1992; Liddle et al., 2001; Springer & Orsbon, 2002). Joanning et al. (1992) compared family systems therapy (FST) and adolescent group treatment to multiple-family drug education groups, but to differentiate the MFGs from the FST condition, they explicitly limited these groups to psychoeducation. Hamilton and colleagues (2001) integrated parent training groups into a broader adolescent substance abuse intervention, but did not include other family members within groups. To date, only one MFG intervention has been rigorously evaluated as a treatment for adolescent substance abusers. At 12 months, Liddle et al. (2001) found that adolescents treated in MFGs experienced clinically significant reductions in drug use. However, when compared to Multidimensional Family Therapy (MDFT) and cognitive-behavioral Adolescent Group Treatment (AGT), those treated in MFGs fared the worst on all measures, including measures of family functioning. Dropout, however, was lower for MFGs than for the AGT condition. Liddle and his colleagues (2001) concluded that MFGs may not provide enough individual attention to families to affect change and cautioned that MFGs should be used in conjunction with other treatment modalities (i.e., individual sessions with adolescents, family therapy). Although the MFG tested by Liddle and colleagues (2001) did not perform as well as MDFT or group treatment, it should be noted that the MFG was used as a stand-alone intervention. Thus, little is known about the potential benefits of adding MFGs to multicomponent interventions, which are rapidly becoming the norm in adolescent substance abuse treatment. Furthermore, these findings need to be replicated to determine if they are robust, or were specific to the only study that has evaluated the outcomes of an MFG.

Potential Benefits of MFGs

Additional studies on the effects of MFGs with adolescent substance abusers are needed for two main reasons. First, treating substance-abusing adolescents in MFGs may be a feasible way that not-for-profit agencies can respond to the demand for family inclusion in adolescent services. That is, to survive in the current managed care environment, these agencies need to efficiently use the time of a limited number of staff members providing services. Thus, if effective family-based group therapy models were available, they may be attractive options to agencies who are struggling to promote family inclusion with existing resources. Dennison (2005) notes that MFGs are time efficient in that therapists can share information with multiple clients at once. Second, using MFGs may also help substance abuse treatment agencies allay some of the current concerns surrounding peer group treatments. Researchers have raised concerns about whether or not iatrogenic effects may occur if adolescents are clustered with other high-risk youth (Dishion & Dodge, 2005; Macgowan & Wagner, 2005; Poulin, Dishion, & Burraston, 2001). Specifically, it is believed that antisocial youth, when aggregated in groups, reinforce each other's antisocial behavior (i.e., peer contagion), which may result in poorer outcomes. Although these findings have yet to be replicated with substance-abusing treatment samples and mixed findings are emerging (Burleson, Kaminer, & Dennis, 2006), treating teens in MFGs could possibly prevent some peer contagion from occurring due to the sheer adult presence in the group. In summary, we argue that MFGs have great potential in treating adolescent substance abusers, because of reduced strain on agency resources and possible prevention of peer contagion effects.

Knowledge Gaps with MFGs

Because of the promise of using MFGs in adolescent's substance abuse treatments, additional research is needed that helps practitioners implement these models. Thus, the purpose of this article is to describe how we implemented MFGs in a not-for-profit agency in the context of a large community effort to expand and enhance adolescent substance abuse treatment. We begin by briefly describing the system of care and the therapy model within which our MFGs are nested. Then, we outline the challenges associated with implementing these MFGs and provide solutions to common implementation issues that others may experience when using similar models.

SYSTEM OF CARE DESCRIPTION

The MFGs considered here were implemented in the context of a 5-year initiative funded by the Substance Abuse and Mental Health Services Administration (SAMHSA), called Strengthening Communities for Youth (SCY). Our community collaboration was located in a two-county area in eastern Iowa, containing semiurban Johnson County (population 100,000+) and rural Iowa County (population 15,000+). The project had six major goals, including providing a continuum of care of services, networking with community partners to expand and enhance adolescent substance abuse treatments, implementing a Web-based management information system to facilitate interagency record sharing, using state-of-the art outreach methods, implementing evidence-based practices, and addressing the association between substance use and violence.

The System of Care before SCY

At the beginning of our collaboration (March 2002), several gaps existed in the community's infrastructure for addressing adolescent substance abuse. First, only one program offered specialized adolescent services, which means that the primary gap in the system of care was the lack of capacity for multiple interventions. One full-time therapist made up the entire adolescent program serving Johnson County youth, and Iowa County youth were served by a generalist substance abuse practitioner that mainly served adults. Other treatment options existed, but teens in these programs were mixed with adults in group therapy, which is problematic as age similarity among group members predicts increased attendance (Kelly, Myers, & Brown, 2005). Second, the system of care lacked residential and intensive outpatient services for adolescents. Thus, the publicly available treatment system was so overwhelmed with the number of referrals from criminal justice that scant time was left for planning to implement new treatment innovations and also focusing on adolescents whose problems had not reached acute severity. Third, this project formalized the drug treatment agency's existing efforts to implement and monitor the outcomes of evidence based practices. Prior to the SCY project, no formal evidence-based curricula were being used consistently in the adolescent program serving this two-county region. Although clinicians in the program had been exposed to evidence-based practices, it was unclear how their exposure to evidence-based practices was being cohesively woven together to form an adolescent treatment approach. This situation was unfortunate, as agencies not only need exposure to research-based interventions, but also need the resources and leadership to sustain and monitor the implementation (Gotham, 2006; Simpson, 2002). Finally, despite published reports on the efficacy of family-based services, very few family-based services were available in the system of care prior to this project (Austin et al., 2005; Waldron, 1997; Williams & Chang, 2000). Thus, a major goal of the Iowa SCY project was to develop and implement a family therapy approach and compare this approach to treatment as usual (i.e., individual and peer group treatment) provided at the agency. In short, the major gaps in the local system of care included the overall lack of capacity, the lack of residential and intensive outpatient services, the uneven implementation of evidence-based practices for adolescent substance abusers, and the lack of family-based services.

To address these major gaps in the system of care for adolescent substance abusers, the SCY collaboration was forged between the University of Iowa's Department of Pediatrics (UI) and the Mid-Eastern Council on Chemical Abuse (MECCA). The UI Department of Pediatrics is nested within a large teaching hospital system in the Carver College of Medicine. MECCA is a licensed, not-for-profit substance abuse provider serving a five-county catchment area in eastern Iowa.

This collaboration addressed existing gaps by funding three additional therapists, adding an intensive outpatient program, developing a centralized assessment center for the two-county service area, and developing a family-based treatment approach (i.e., SOFT). The remainder of this article focuses on the latter task of implementing the SOFT model, with an emphasis on challenges faced with our MFGs.

STRENGTHS-ORIENTED FAMILY THERAPY

SOFT Description, Development, and Implementation

SOFT blends solution-focused family therapy, family communication skills training in MFGs, and targeted case management for adolescents who abuse substances (Hall, Smith, & Williams, 2008; Smith & Hall, 2008). We start with a rigorous family assessment procedure culminating in a protocol called Strengths Oriented Referral for Teens (SORT) (Smith & Hall, 2007), where results from a structured substance abuse and mental health assessment are presented to the teen and parent using Motivational Interviewing and solution-focused techniques (Berg & Miller, 1992; Miller & Rollnick, 2002). If the family engages in SOFT treatment after the SORT session they then progress through three stages of treatment: (1) engagement and initial strengths assessment, (2) development and implementation of a solution plan, and (3) monitoring and refining of goals until termination. Adolescents and parents are encouraged to attend counseling sessions together, unless high conflict precludes productive family sessions. In addition to the conjoint family sessions, families attend weekly MFGs. Families also receive case management on an as-needed basis. For a comprehensive description of the therapy model, see Hall et al. (2008).

SOFT multiple-family group. The SOFT MFG blends solution-focused group interaction, family communications skills training, and cognitive-behavioral therapy specific to substance abuse treatment. Group topics include (1) giving and receiving positive feedback, (2) listening assertively, (3) giving and receiving constructive criticism, (4) coping with using peers, (5) solving problems, (6) solving family problems, (7) building healthy relationships and fighting fairly, (8) managing stress, (9) managing anger, and (10) preventing future substance use and abuse by the adolescent. The groups are structured and task oriented, and the basic format includes a brief check-in (i.e., solution-focused questions presuming change, scaling questions), a short lecture and discussion about a skills topic (i.e., rationale for activities, describe topic), and role-playing. Despite the structure, groups are highly interactive. For example, we encourage peer support and normalize situations for families, which are proposed curative features of group therapy (Yalom & Leszcz, 2005). Families complete feedback forms to comment on the usefulness of the groups.

Rationale for SOFT development. Two main reasons influenced our decision to develop and test SOFT. First, as mentioned before, the local system of care did not have any family-based adolescent substance abuse treatment options. Second, we wanted to test widely popular therapy techniques that are part of the SOFT model (i.e., solution-focused therapy, strengths-based treatments) that have rarely been subject to sound empirical validation (Allen, Donohue, Griffin, Ryan, & Turner, 2003; Selekman, 1997; Staudt, Howard, & Drake, 2001). SOFT differs from other family-based models by including formal strengths assessments, MFGs, and heavy emphasis on solution-focused language in all phases of treatment. As previously mentioned, few researchers have evaluated the effects of MFGs with adolescent substance abusers.

Initial development of SOFT MFGs. The two main therapists providing SOFT at MECCA were instrumental in developing the MFG content. After receiving mentoring by the lead developers on how to write replicable treatment sessions, they collaborated in the development of new group activities and adaptation of activities from a skills training model for use with pregnant and parenting teens, as well as with rural secondary students (Hall, 1995). This process of close collaboration with community practitioners is recommended in the National Institutes of Health (NIH) stage model of behavioral therapy development, as it capitalizes on the creativity of practitioners to complement the expertise of clinical researchers (Rounsaville, Carroll, & Onken, 2001). Both therapists that helped develop the SOFT MFGs were highly committed to the project and remained with us for the entire 5-year duration of the project. This commitment may have been partially due to a sense of ownership we fostered by including them in the intervention development process.

Preliminary outcomes. Although MFGs have been used extensively by social workers, their effects have rarely been evaluated (Dennison, 1999, 2005). As part of a clinical trial, we evaluated the 6-month outcomes for adolescents who received SOFT. We found that adolescents receiving SOFT experienced significant reductions in drug use and drug-related problems (Smith, Hall, Williams, An, & Gotman, 2006). Although these results are for the overall SOFT model, it should be noted that the MFGs make up two thirds of the prescribed content of SOFT. Our current research is focusing on the impact SOFT had on family functioning and mental health outcomes.

IMPLEMENTING MULTIPLE-FAMILY GROUPS

Implementation Challenges

We faced several challenges in implementing the MFGs within our system of care. Implementation challenges occurred at the external, organizational, and individual levels (Gotham, 2006). External factors affecting implementation efforts include state policies and other macro issues that influence service provision. Organizational factors include support from management, organizational stress, and organization communication. Finally, individual-level factors that influence service implementation include staff attitudes, skills, and adaptability. At an intersection between the external and organizational levels, we found that implementing MFGs met the agency's need of providing service hours dictated by state licensure requirements within parameters of existing staff resources. At the external level, we found that implementation was influenced by geographic location of clients, with urban locations better suited to conducting group therapy. Organizational-level factors that influenced implementation included supervision structure and agency staffing patterns. Individual-level factors influencing the implementation of MFGs included therapist group facilitation skills, therapist perceptions that family members would not attend MFGs, and therapist concerns surrounding always having parents present in groups.

External-Level Challenges

Meeting state licensure standards. The SOFT MFGs were born out of a compromise with our partners at MECCA, a community not-for-profit substance abuse treatment agency. Our original plan was to deliver all of the SOFT intervention content in conjoint family sessions, but we discovered that this plan would be logistically impossible due to problems with meeting agency licensure standards for required service hours. That is, adolescents receiving intensive outpatient therapy at MECCA were required to receive a minimum of six service hours per week. If one therapist provided six service hours per week to a single family, case loads would have been small and the program would have been difficult to sustain. Thus, to approximate these weekly service hours, we implemented a weekly, 2-hour multiple-family group to complement a weekly 2-hour conjoint family session. This process finding underscored the utility of MFGs in agency settings, that are not only facing limited staff resources, but also required to comply with licensure standards that affect what treatments they implement.

Rural service provision. The geographic location of the clients' homes was an additional external factor influencing MFG implementation. Specifically, we found that rural clients were less likely to participate in MFGs when compared to their urban counterparts. Although some rural families commuted to our urban office to receive services, this was not the norm. Thus, traveling long distances to receive MFG services was likely a barrier. Unfortunately, because of uneven case flow, we were unable to offer open MFGs in rural locations. During our project, we modified the MFG activities and delivered it in in-home conjoint family sessions to rural families. Because of this process finding, we believe that technological solutions such as live videoconferencing should be pursued as potential solutions that may facilitate rural adolescent substance abusers to participate in such groups.

Organizational-Level Challenges

Initial training and ongoing supervision. In addition to brief training workshops, we found that ongoing monitoring efforts are vital to the success of implementing our new program. In our context, the organization was supportive of allowing the intervention developers to provide initial trainings on the MFG model, as well as ongoing clinical supervision. Simpson (2002) identified various stages of implementation that we use here to guide our discussion of initial development and ongoing monitoring of the SOFT MFG. The stages include exposure, implementation and practice.[1]

Simpson (2002) defines *exposure training* as the first stage in implementing a program in clinical practice. We initially trained therapists on the principles of solution-focused therapy, as well as on basic group processes we wanted to use in MFG therapy. For example, in activities where adolescents are role-playing communication skills, we instructed therapists to match adolescents with other adults in the group. This technique was presented as a useful tool to build cohesiveness between group members and at the same time allow communication skills training to proceed uninterrupted by ongoing family conflicts between parents and teens.

After initial training on the model and the development of all the sessions, we entered Simpson's (2002) *implementation* stage. In this stage, exploratory use and mastery of the content are the primary goals. We decided to have therapists co-facilitate MFGs when they were first learning the techniques and intervention content, as we felt that this would allow them to master the session content without sacrificing attention to the complex group dynamics of MFGs. All early sessions were recorded and reviewed on a weekly basis in clinical supervision.

After mastering the content, we moved into Simpson's (2002) *practice* stage, when the MFGs became integrated into the services offered within the adolescent therapy program. A lead developer provided weekly supervision to therapists, which focused on proper use of the session content as well as focusing on group dynamics.

Although the development and implementation process went smoothly, we experienced one major challenge within our overall strategy. Specifically, although supervision with the lead developer was intensive during the exposure stage, barriers emerged that limited access to ongoing supervision during the practice stage. Ongoing supervision with the lead developer became part of the agency's regularly scheduled group clinical supervision, which also involved lengthy discussions of the adolescents' treatment progress (called continued stay reviews). In these continued stay reviews, client progress is monitored to ensure that services are adequate at the current level of care. As part of the documentation process, supervisors approve of a clinician's overall justification to continue services. In our situation, continued stay reviews were necessary to obtain reimbursement from state and private funding sources, and were completed by reviewing each client using the American Society for Addictions Medicine's (ASAM) criteria (Mee-Lee, Gartner, Miller, Shulman, & Wilford, 2001). The agency need for completing continued stay reviews during clinical supervision took away from dedicated time to continue processing how the MFGs were running. In short, supervision was mainly focused on client progress at the individual level, and the status of the group became one among many agenda items during group supervision. Continued stay reviews would take up most of group supervision time when caseloads ballooned, which forced the MFG lead developer attending these supervision meetings to make extra efforts during group supervision to address the quality of the MFG services. For example, we developed an agenda for group supervision meetings, so we focused our attention on group process issues such as group cohesion, leadership within the groups, and whether or not any members were not participating. Having a list of standard questions to ask therapists about the group's functioning prompted our attention to these important issues. Additionally, to supplement group supervision, spot-checks on audio recordings or live observation of groups are recommended.

Rotating group coverage. An additional organizational-level challenge we experienced was that MECCA ensured continuous group coverage by using two different SOFT therapists. That is, the two SOFT therapists facilitated the group on a biweekly basis, and it is unclear what impact this had on the group process or the quality of the group. On one hand, because therapists had families on their caseloads attending the MFGs, rotating coverage may have provided better continuity versus simply having a different group facilitator altogether. Also, families may have benefited by exposure to different therapists who may have different styles including fresh perspectives helpful to families reaching sticking points. On the other hand, having two therapists cover the group may have interrupted the continuity of the group. For example, at the very beginning of each group there is a brief review of the previous session and the previous week's therapeutic assignments. To address this issue, therapists frequently consulted with each other on critical events occurring within the group.

Individual-Level Challenges

At the individual level, we identified some challenges with the clinicians facilitating the MFGs. First, clinicians needed additional training on making groups more interactive. Second, there was concern that family members would not get involved or attend MFGs if they were offered. Additionally, therapists voiced concerns about including parents in all group sessions and felt that adolescents would be less likely to share about drug-use opportunities and continued use.

Individual therapy in a group setting. One issue that we identified early on in supervision was that therapists favored using extended check-ins with individual clients and were not integrating other group members in ways that build cohesion and foster peer support. Additional training with therapists focused on including multiple members' comments in tandem, as well as on the importance of family-to-family support as a potential curative factor operating within MFGs. That is, directive methods for managing group conversations were modeled and reviewed in addition to providing the rationale for why family-to-family support is so crucial. For example, therapists were taught to track how often conversation flowed only from the member to therapist. Audiotape reviews are particularly helpful for demonstrating this, because rather than relying on vague descriptions of this phenomenon, clinicians can hear and better operationalize the level of member-to-member interaction.

Parental attendance. Prior to the implementation of MFGs, some clinicians in the agency doubted whether parents would actually attend such groups and be involved in their adolescents' treatment. Our experience was that parental attendance was the rule rather than the exception. Families, on average, completed about 60% of the group content in our SOFT intervention, but, consistent with other published reports on high overall dropout in substance abuse treatment, completion by our families was highly variable (Smith et al., 2006). Our completion rate reflects some dropout but also how some youth were unable to come to group due to competing prosocial activities on their schedules (i.e., sports, vacations). In other studies with family interventions, parental attendance at groups was also high (Dennis et al., 2004). In short, the majority of parents were able to attend these groups, and overall completion was consistent with other published treatment studies.

We also found that teens rarely said they did not want their parents to come to sessions. Out of 210 adolescents that were eligible for participation in the current study (and thus MFGs), we know of only one adolescent that actively refused to participate in family-based treatment. This adolescent was reassigned to the adolescent–peer group treatment condition.

In summary, we find that initial concerns that parents would not attend treatment seemed to be largely unfounded. We believe that parental participation was maximized in our MFGs due to patental inclusion in agency intakes and the scheduling of groups in the evening, which usually didn't conflict with parents' work schedules. Our family-based assessments were designed to empathize with parents and, if applicable, educate them to the treatment needs of their adolescents (Smith & Hall, 2007). During these family-based assessments we also oriented family members to the purpose, topics, and duration of the MFGs. In short, we feel that parents will attend MFGs if they are included in the treatment process early, are oriented to treatment needs and their role in problem resolution, and if groups do not conflict with work schedules.

Teen-only MFG sessions. Therapists implementing the SOFT MFGs were uneasy about always including parents in groups. Two main reasons were offered by therapists. First, therapists felt that teens participating in MFGs would not freely discuss their substance use and family issues when their and other teens' parents were present. Second, therapists argued that they needed additional time to build rapport with the adolescents and wanted this time built within the structure of the MFGs.

We as researchers were initially concerned with holding teen-only group sessions, because our original goals were to compare a family-based intervention with a teen-focused treatment as usual condition. As we thought that some of the mechanisms affecting overall treatment outcomes were embedded within group therapy (i.e., deviancy training, meeting other participants to use drugs after group), we initially resisted developing an adolescent-only group session within the SOFT model. That is, we assumed that some negative processes putatively present in adolescent-only group therapy would work against overall treatment outcomes, and if we added this component to SOFT, it would weaken the comparison. Additionally, when adding a teen-only group to the MFG sessions was proposed, the therapists resisted the idea of scripting this session and voiced preferences that this session be an interactive open session.

Ultimately, we compromised and developed an adolescent-only group. However, we built it within the logical flow (and structure) of the SOFT MFG activities. In the fifth group, adolescents attend alone and therapists are permitted to do an extended check-in and group discussion around the theme of what changes they have observed in their parents during treatment and whether they've used refusal skills, which were taught in the previous group. During this group, therapists also follow up on whether they have asked a peer with whom they have previously used drugs (i.e., previous week's homework) to provide them with support to remain abstinent. We thought that this conversation may be more productive when parents were absent. If a good group discussion ensues, therapists are allowed to stick with it as long as it remains focused on the skills, the previous week's homework, and family themes in the intervention. However, if the discussion ends quickly, therapists complete a planned problem-solving activity with the teens. This activity overlaps with a family problem-solving activity that occurs in the next session when parents attend the MFG.

This concern highlights what we feel is a broader issue encountered when implementing MFGs in agencies that have historically been adolescent focused. That is, therapists appear to need assistance and reassurance that confidentiality issues that arise in family-based treatments are easily overcome. Perhaps central to the problem of adding parents in adolescent substance abuse treatment is the issue of managing multiple relationships. Here we found that therapists seemed to perceive that most adolescents want to limit information given to parents about their drug use and other behaviors. However, we found that adolescents in treatment were remarkably open with their parents, and that most of our concerns were based on unfounded assumptions that teens would always want to limit information to parents. Specifically, when teens were directly asked about whether we could share information about their substance use with their parents, the majority said we could. This is not to say we do not have some adolescents that did not want their therapists to share information with their parents. To protect adolescents' legal rights to confidentiality, we train therapists how to directly ask adolescents what was permissible to share, as well as how to explore with adolescents the potential benefits and consequences of disclosing sensitive information to their parents.

Therapists' perceptions that adolescents were guarding information in MFGs may have also been influenced by some fundamental misunderstandings of the model and of group process. For example, therapists during supervision would frequently describe adolescents as "resistant" or "lacking ownership of their behaviors" when they were not disclosing continued substance use to the group that had been discussed with the therapists individually or in family sessions. In supervision we reframe this as a group process issue and begin asking questions about how long the teen in question has been attending the group and how cohesive the group is.

The fact that therapists wanted an open processing session with only the adolescents may also reflect their lack of familiarity with structured MFGs. We knew that most of their group experience was with open groups where the emphasis was only on group discussion. An essential part of group leadership in MFGs, however, is providing structure for the group process to unfold (Dennison, 2005). We argue that adolescents can change substance-using behaviors when these behaviors are addressed directly and indirectly. For example, when we complete structured family communication exercises in the MFG we are indirectly addressing substance use through the process of strengthening the family system. Although we provide a rationale to families regarding how all exercises are related to the overall goal of reducing the adolescents' substance use, it appeared that therapists like to address substance use issues head on through discussion of the use itself. Thus, therapists need reassurance that substance use reduction can also be accomplished indirectly via working through families in groups, and they need reminders that group structure is an important element necessary for developing working groups.

MULTIPLE-FAMILY GROUP IMPLEMENTATION RECOMMENDATIONS

Based on the implementation experiences described here, we conclude with some general recommendations for implementing MFGs in adolescent substance abuse treatment.

- To facilitate buy-in from therapists, stress their importance in developing activities for groups. If implementing an existing evidence-based MFG, enlist therapists to make appropriate adaptations to meet the needs of their diverse clientele.
- In training therapists, model the integration of comments by multiple group members into a cohesive group process. Discourage therapists from focusing too much attention on single participants at the expense of the overall group.
- During clinical supervision, make sure that group process issues are discussed in addition to the individual progress. Ask questions about the level of cohesion for the group, about which members the therapists consider to be leaders, and if any members are not actively participating in group. Consider developing a list of standard questions to address in clinical supervision about how groups are functioning. Use audio recordings or live supervision to ensure that the group is running smoothly.
- We recommend using no more than two therapists to cover an open MFG. Additionally, if two therapists share group coverage, encourage regular communication about any critical events in group and what content was covered.
- To increase family participation in MFGs we recommend including parents or guardians in initial assessments. Family assessment protocols are available (Dishion, Nelson, & Kavanagh, 2003; Smith & Hall, 2007). We also recommend conducting groups during evening hours when parents and guardians can attend.
- Address therapists' assumptions with sensitivity by reframing their concerns as being grounded in their desire to help clients. Encourage them to check out their practice assumptions with actual client feedback (i.e., data). Then, provide reassurances in the following areas:
  - Reassure therapists that parents do indeed attend MFGs. Review published rates of parental attendance with therapists.
  - Reassure therapists that treatment satisfaction among clients is not necessarily sacrificed when group structure is high or when adolescents are mixed with their parents. In the current study, overall treatment satisfaction among adolescents was higher for the SOFT intervention than for controls who received less structured group therapy (Hall et al., 2008).
  - Reassure therapists that confidentiality issues, if handled sensitively, can be readily overcome, and that many adolescents are perfectly comfortable with sharing information with their parents.

CONCLUSION

MFG treatment models are promising interventions for use in adolescent substance abuse treatment facilities. These group approaches are time-efficient models that can address external demands to include family members in the treatment process. Implementation issues identified in this article can be successfully overcome, which is encouraging because two independent investigators found significant reductions in substance use among adolescents receiving MFG content. As this implementation experience may not generalize to all practice settings, research should continue to focus on the implementation of MFGs. Additionally, empirical work is desperately needed on the treatment outcomes of adolescent substance abusers treated in MFGs, as well as on the mechanisms within MFGs that foster clinical change. Thus, due to the feasibility of treating adolescent substance abusers with MFGs in community practice settings, we are hopeful that researchers will collaborate with these community agencies to evaluate the impact of this clinically important component.

ACKNOWLEDGMENT

The development of this article was supported by the Substance Abuse and Mental Health Services Administration (SAMHSA: CSAT TI13354). Dr. Smith is now Assistant Professor in the School of Social Work, University of Illinois. Dr. Hall is now Dean of The University of Alabama School of Social Work.

NOTE

1. Simpson (2002) also defined a stage called "adoption," during which decisions are made about whether to use an intervention. In our context, agreements between researchers and the community not-for-profit agency about trying new interventions were made prior to implementation efforts when we collaborated on writing the grant supporting these services. Nevertheless, therapist commitment to the model (and adoption) was facilitated by enlisting their help in developing sessions, as previously described.

REFERENCES

Allen, M., Donohue, W. A., Griffin, A., Ryan, D., & Turner, M. M. (2003). Comparing the influence of parents and peers on the choice to use drugs. *Criminal Justice & Behavior, 30*(2), 163–186.

Austin, A. M., Macgowan, M. J., & Wagner, E. F. (2005). Effective family-based interventions for adolescents with substance abuse problems: A systematic review. *Research on Social Work Practice, 15*(2), 67–83.

Berg, I. K., & Miller, S. D. (1992). *Working with a problem drinker: A solution-focused approach*. New York: W.W. Norton.

Bronfenbrenner, U. (1986). Ecology of the family as a context for human development: Research perspectives. *Developmental Psychology, 22*(6), 723–742.

Burleson, J. A., Kaminer, Y., & Dennis, M. L. (2006). Absence of iatrogenic or contagion effects in adolescent group therapy: Findings from the Cannabis Youth Treatment (CYT) study. *American Journal on Addictions*, (Suppl 1) *15*, 4–15.

Dennis, M. L., Godley, S. H., Diamond, G., Tims, F. M., Babor, T., Donaldson, J., et al. (2004). The Cannabis Youth Treatment (CYT) Study: Main findings from two randomized trials. *Journal of Substance Abuse Treatment, 27*(3), 197–213.

Dennison, S. T. (1999). Multiple-family groups: Practice implications for the 21st century. *Journal of Family Social Work, 3*(3), 29–51.

Dennison, S. T. (2005). *A multiple family group therapy program for at-risk adolescents and their families*. Springfield, IL: Charles C Thomas.

Dishion, T. J., & Dodge, K. A. (2005). Peer contagion in interventions for children and adolescents: Moving towards an understanding of the ecology and dynamics of change. *Journal of Abnormal Child Psychology, 33*(3), 395–400.

Dishion, T. J., Nelson, S. E., & Kavanagh, K. (2003). The family check-up with high-risk young adolescents: Preventing early-onset substance use by parent monitoring. *Behavior Therapy, 34*(4), 553–571.

Gotham, H. J. (2006). Advancing the implementation of evidence-based practices into clinical practice: How do we get there from here? *Clinical Psychology: Research and Practice, 37*(6), 606–613.

Hall, J. A. (1995). *PALS strength training: Improving positive adolescent life skills and preventing risky behaviors and situations (student handbook)*. Unpublished manuscript, University of Iowa, Iowa City, IA.

Hall, J. A., Smith, D. C., & Williams, J. K. (2008). Strengths Oriented Family Therapy (SOFT): A manual guided treatment for substance-involved teens and their families. In C. W. Lecroy (Ed.), *Handbook of evidence-based treatment manuals for children and adolescents* (2nd ed., pp. 491–545). New York: Oxford University Press.

Hamilton, N. L., Brantley, L. B., Tims, F. M., Angelovich, N., & McDougall, B. (2001). *Family support network for adolescent cannabis users, Cannabis Youth Treatment (CYT) series, volume 3*. Silver Spring, MD: Substance Abuse and Mental Health Services Administration.

Joanning, H., Quinn, W., Thomas, F., & Mullen, R. (1992). Treating adolescent drug abuse: A comparison of family systems therapy, group therapy, and family drug education. *Journal of Marital & Family Therapy, 18*(4), 345–356.

Kelly, J. F., Myers, M. G., & Brown, S. A. (2005). The effects of age composition of 12-step groups on adolescent 12-step participation and substance use outcome. *Journal of Child and Adolescent Substance Abuse, 15*(1), 63–72.

Liddle, H. A. (2004). Family-based therapies for adolescent alcohol and drug use: Research contributions and future research needs. *Addiction, 99*(Suppl 2), 76–92.

Liddle, H. A., Dakof, G. A., Parker, K., Diamond, G. S., Barrett, K., & Tejeda, M. (2001). Multidimensional family therapy for adolescent drug abuse: Results of a randomized clinical trial. *American Journal of Drug & Alcohol Abuse, 27*(4), 651–688.

Liddle, H. A., Rowe, C. L., Gonzalez, A., Henderson, C. E., Dakof, G. A., & Greenbaum, P. E. (2006). Changing provider practices, program environment, and improving outcomes by transporting multidimensional family therapy to an adolescent drug treatment setting. *American Journal on Addictions, 15*, 102–112.

Macgowan, M. J., & Wagner, E. F. (2005). Iatrogenic effects of group treatment on adolescents with conduct disorder and substance use problems: A review of the literature and a presentation of a model. *Journal of Evidence-Based Social Work*, 2(1/2), 79–90.

Mee-Lee, D., Gartner, L., Miller, M. M., Shulman, G., & Wilford, B. (2001). *Patient Placement Criteria, second edition-revised (ASAM PPC-2R)*. Annapolis Junction, MD: American Society of Addiction Medicine.

Meezan, W., & O'Keefe, M. (1998). Evaluating the effectiveness of multifamily group therapy in child abuse and neglect. *Research on Social Work Practice*, 8(3), 330–353.

Miller, W. R., & Rollnick, S. (2002). *Motivational Interviewing: Preparing people for change* (2nd ed.). New York: Guilford Press.

Poulin, F., Dishion, T. J., & Burraston, B. (2001). 3-Year iatrogenic effects associated with aggregating high-risk adolescents in cognitive-behavioral preventive interventions. *Applied Developmental Science*, 5(4), 214–224.

Rounsaville, B. J., Carroll, K. M., & Onken, L. S. (2001). A stage model of behavioral therapies research: Getting started and moving on from stage I. *Clinical Psychology: Science and Practice*, 8(2), 133–142.

Selekman, M. D. (1997). *Solution-focused therapy with children: Harnessing family strengths for systemic change*. New York: Guilford Press.

Simpson, D. D. (2002). A conceptual framework for transferring research to practice. *Journal of Substance Abuse Treatment*, 22, 171–182.

Smith, D. C., & Hall, J. A. (2007). Strengths-Oriented Referral for Teens (SORT): Giving balanced feedback to teens and families. *Health & Social Work*, 32(1), 69–72.

Smith, D. C., & Hall, J. A. (2008). Strengths-oriented family therapy for adolescents with substance abuse problems. *Social Work* 53(2), 185–188.

Smith, D. C., Hall, J. A., Williams, J., An, H., & Gotman, N. (2006). Comparative efficacy of family and group treatment for adolescent substance abuse. *American Journal on Addictions*, (Suppl 1)(6), 131–136.

Springer, D. W., & Orsbon, S. H. (2002). Families helping families: Implementing a multifamily therapy group with substance-abusing adolescents. *Health & Social Work*, 27(3), 204–207.

Staudt, M., Howard, M. O., & Drake, B. (2001). The operationalization, implementation and effectiveness of the strengths perspective: A review of empirical studies. *Journal of Social Service Research*, 27(3), 1–21.

Steinberg, L., Lamborn, S. D., Darling, N., Mounts, N. S., & Dornbusch, S. M. (1994). Over time adjustment and competence among adolescents from authoritative, authoritarian, indulgent, and neglectful families. *Child Development*, 65, 754–770.

Waldron, H. B. (1997). Adolescent substance abuse and family therapy outcome: A review of randomized trials. In T. H. Ollendick & R. J. Prinz (Eds.), *Advances in clinical child psychology* (pp. 199–234). New York: Plenum Press.

Williams, R. J., & Chang, S. Y. (2000). A comprehensive and comparative review of adolescent substance abuse treatment outcome. *Clinical Psychology-Science & Practice*, 7(2), 138–166.

Yalom, I. D., & Leszcz, M. (2005). *The theory and practice of group psychotherapy*. New York: Basic Books.

"I'm not lazy; it's just that I learn differently": Development and Implementation of a Manualized School-Based Group for Students with Learning Disabilities

FAYE MISHNA

University of Toronto, Factor-Inwentash Faculty of Social Work, Toronto, Ontario, Canada

BARBARA MUSKAT

The Hospital for Sick Children, Toronto, Ontario, Canada

JUDITH WIENER

Ontario Institute for Studies in Education at the University of Toronto, Ontario, Canada

In this article the authors present the implementation and pilot evaluation of an innovative manualized school-based group for middle-school students with a learning disability (LD). The group was one component of a school-based intervention that was a collaboration of university-based researchers, children's mental health, and education. Interviews were held with selected students, their parents, and teachers to obtain their views of the group. Preliminary findings suggest that the group improved students' knowledge of their LD, increased their ability to ask for help and self-advocate, and enhanced their confidence. The group leaders found the manualized group beneficial and offered recommendations for change. Practice principles in providing group for students with LD are offered.

INTRODUCTION

During the past decade there has been a proliferation in the literature on the number and types of group treatment approaches for children and adolescents, in a wide range of settings (Lomonaco, Scheidlinger, & Aronson, 2000). Anecdotal and research evidence supports the benefits of group interventions for individuals of all ages (Bratton, Ray, Rhine, & Jones, 2005; Hoag & Burlingame, 1997; Page, Weiss, & Lietaer, 2001; Weisz, Weiss, Han, Granger, & Morton, 1995), and specifically for children and adolescents (Cramer-Azima, 2002). Moreover, group intervention remains the treatment of choice for children and youth (Cramer-Azima, 2002), in particular for problems with peer relationships (Lomonaco et al., 2000).

Although many individuals with learning disabilities (LD) do not have psychosocial difficulties (Morrison & Cosden, 1997), students with LD are more likely than their peers without LD to develop psychosocial problems (Cosden, 2001; McNamara, Willoughby, Chalmers, & YLC-CURA, 2005). Cognitive deficits, inherent to LD, put students at risk of inadequate academic performance and failure (Pearl & Bay, 1999), which is associated with poor adjustment, including life-course-impairing psychiatric disorders and compromised social and vocational functioning (Cosden, 2001; Maag & Reid, 2006; Margalit & Al-Yagon, 2002; Morrison & Cosden, 1997; Offord, Boyle, & Racine, 1990; Pearl & Bay, 1999; Svetaz, Ireland, & Blum, 2000). Evidence suggests that approximately 25% to 30% of students with LD are rejected by peers in comparison to 8% to 16% of their peers without LD (Greenham, 1999) and that they are more likely to be bullied by their peers (Nabuzoka, 2003).

In this article, we present a manualized school-based group intervention for students with LD. Despite modifications that may be required due to their cognitive deficits, many children and adolescents with LD fit the criteria for and can benefit from group treatment (Mishna, 1996a; Mishna & Muskat, 2004a; Shechtman & Pastor, 2005).

Evidence-based group work practice involves using the best available evidence to design, pilot, and modify new approaches; carry out full-scale evaluations with the collaboration of practitioners and researchers; obtain feedback from members of the target population; and disseminate results (Galinsky, Terzian, & Fraser, 2006; Pollio, 2002). In this article we present the development and implementation of an innovative manualized school-based group for middle-school students with LD (Muskat, 2004). The group was one component of a school-based intervention that was a collaboration of university-based researchers and children's mental health and education practitioners. Consistent with the view that "formative evaluation including process observation is essential to revising a program" (Farrell, Meyer, & Dahlberg, 1996, p. 19), the group approach was modified based on the promising results of a previous study that examined a school-based program for students with LD (Mishna & Muskat, 2004b).

The aim of the larger school-based intervention was to enhance the environment in which the students function and, within this more supportive context, offer group treatment. The intervention program was innovative in that there were multiple targets for change including the students with LD, their parents, teachers, and peers without LD, and there were unique components, including the group presented in this article. The school-based group for students constituted the treatment provided to the participating students with LD and is the focus of this article. Objectives of the group component were to (1) increase the students' knowledge and understanding of LD, (2) increase their awareness and knowledge of their learning strengths and deficits, and (3) increase their ability to advocate for themselves.

The objectives of the overall research were to (1) evaluate the effectiveness of the program, incorporating individual, social, and environmental levels; (2) contribute to knowledge about factors that influence adjustment of students with LD; and (3) disseminate this information to educators, parents, and others who work with children who have LD. We present preliminary results from interviews with students who participated in the research including the group treatment, and their parents and teachers, on their experience and views of the group component of the overall research project. The two other components, which are not presented in this article, comprised workshops on LD for peers without LD, parents, and teachers and consultation for teachers of students in the group.

In this article, we review psychosocial difficulties associated with LD, demonstrate the applicability of group interventions for students with LD, and describe the development and implementation of a manualized school-based group that builds on previous research. Preliminary results from interviews with students who participated in the group, as well as from their teachers and parents, are presented, followed by practice implications.

STUDENTS WITH LEARNING DISABILITIES

Typically, support for students with LD addresses academic or remedial skills, with less attention paid to social skills, and there is a notable lack of interventions targeting emotional problems (Shechtman & Pastor, 2005). Although factors such as LD subtype, temperament, and co-existing conditions, as well as family characteristics influence the adjustment of students with LD, the school environment can promote or inhibit academic and psychosocial adjustment (Dishion & Kavanagh, 2000; Pavri & Hegwer-DiVita, 2006). Indeed, LD need not lead to unfavorable adult outcomes (Freeman, Stoch, Chan, & Hutchinson, 2004). An individual's intrinsic traits in combination with familial, educational, and social factors determine academic, vocational, and relational outcomes (Cosden, Brown, & Elliott, 2002; Sorensen et al., 2003). Hence, individually focused interventions are insufficient, as they do not address the ecological conditions that influence adjustment (Bronfenbrenner, 1986, 1994; Elbaum & Vaughn, 2001; Germain & Bloom, 1999; Wiener, 2003).

It is essential to address these factors and the milieu in which children function, to enhance protective factors and offset risk factors (Morrison & Cosden, 1997; Vaughn, Elbaum, & Boardman, 2001). An aim of intervention is to ameliorate risk factors and promote protective factors associated with adjustment of individuals who have LD (Morrison & Cosden, 1997). Factors can be internal or external to an individual and are due to interactions between individuals and domains within their environment. School and family support can protect students with LD from negative school and peer experiences (Svetaz et al., 2000) and help students deal with such experiences (Margalit, 2004). Other protective factors are self-esteem, understanding one's LD, positive relationships with peers and teachers (Wiener, 2002), and high school graduation (Cosden, 2001; Morrison & Cosden, 1997). Poor social skills; noncompliant, aggressive, or disruptive behavior; poor academic achievement; and language impairment (Pearl & Bay, 1999) increase the likelihood that a student with LD will have psychosocial problems.

Although students with LD often perceive their general self-concept similarly to peers without LD, they tend to have lower academic self-concept (Stone & May, 2002). They are more prone to adjustment problems (Al-Yagon & Mikulincer, 2004), and their school dropout rate is higher (Sinclair, Christenson, Evelo, & Hurley, 1998). The transition to middle and high school can affect many children adversely (Kuperminc, Leadbeater, & Blatt, 2001). This move can prove especially difficult for students with LD, who are at risk of losing motivation or of developing antisocial behaviors (Simons-Morton, Crump, Haynie, & Saylor, 1999).

GROUP TREATMENT FOR CHILDREN AND ADOLESCENTS

Group treatment provides a peer group for children and adolescents who are alienated and fosters social competence, through improving social skills, decreasing the sense of isolation, and building self-esteem through acceptance by peers and helping others (Hoag & Burlingame; Malekoff, 2004; Scheidlinger & Aronson, 1991). Other benefits include the opportunity to experience support and safety among peers. The miniature real-life situation in group treatment, through which members can learn about and change behaviors, is consistent with an approach to teaching behavior that takes advantage of naturally occurring incidents, considered "teachable moments" (Gresham, Sugai, & Horner, 2001; Malekoff, 2004; Mishna, 1996a, b; Mishna & Muskat, 2004a; Scheidlinger & Aronson, 1991). This is particularly salient as children are more apt to learn from social interactions with peers than from adults (McIntosh & Vaughn, 1993).

School-Based Group Interventions

Increasingly, a wide variety of group interventions, such as psychoeducation, task-oriented, and counseling groups that address diverse problem areas, are offered within schools (Akos, 2000; Berkovitz, 1989; DeLucia-Waack, 2000). With schools the foremost setting for social development, school-based programs reach students who may not otherwise access service or who are at risk of school dropout (Dishion & Kavanagh, 2000; Meyer & Farrell, 1998; Weist, Nabors, Myers, & Armbruster, 2000). There are a number of advantages to school-based groups as a result of the ongoing contact that is possible among members and/or leaders. These include the opportunity to clarify issues, to reassure members about problems that emerge in sessions, and to be able to comment on such issues as members' positive changes (Berkovitz, 1989). Berkovitz (1989) maintains, "the use of group counselling in the schools represents one of the important preventive mental health measures for children and adolescents" (p. 119). A meta-analysis of 64 school-based programs between 1975 and 1997 that addressed their impact on the self-concept of students with LD found that school-based counseling was more helpful for middle and high school than elementary-age students whereas academically based programs were more helpful for elementary students (Elbaum & Vaughn, 2001).

Groups for Students with LD

Evidence indicates that various group treatment approaches are effective for students with LD (Shechtman & Pastor, 2005). Along with the general benefits of group, specific advantages of group treatment for children and adolescents with LD include the opportunity to be with similar peers who are struggling with common problems and to discuss their LD and its impact. The approximation of group treatment to real life is considered particularly important for students with LD (Berg & Wages, 1982), as their social difficulties can be addressed as they occur, in an accepting environment that is adapted to members' cognitive difficulties and strengths (Carabine & Downton, 2000; Mishna, 1996a, b).

GROUP TREATMENT APPROACH

Theoretical Foundations

The group approach employed in the current study is unique in integrating several theoretical approaches to address issues common to students with LD. The group is guided by evidence that positive outcomes for individuals with LD are associated with such factors as coming to terms with one's LD, self-awareness, persistence, goal setting, and having positive support systems (Miller, 2002; Raskind, Goldberg, Higgins, & Herman, 1999). Programs designed to increase self-determination are considered best practice for students with disabilities (Wehmeyer, Field, Doren, Jones, & Mason, 2004). Self-determination activities are typically targeted to adolescents, yet younger students must acquire foundational skills for self-determination (Mason, Field, & Sawilowsky, 2004; Palmer & Wehmeyer, 2003). Self-advocacy, one component of self-determination, comprises knowledge of one's learning strengths and difficulties, awareness of one's rights and responsibilities, awareness of accommodations needed, and the ability to communicate one's learning needs and required accommodations (Merchant & Gajar, 1997). Students with LD often report that their parents and teachers do not discuss their LD with them, yet such conversations are vital for self-determination (Eisenman & Tascione, 2002). Thus the content in this group model is focused on increasing the students' understanding of their LD and self-advocacy skills.

The group is also guided by a combination of self0psychology (Kohut, 1984), mutual aid (Gitterman & Shulman, 1994), and interpersonal group theory (Yalom & Lescz, 2005). Self-psychology theory posits that an individual's basic needs center on empathic connections with others (Kohut, 1984), fostered in group therapy, which provides an opportunity to feel similar to others. *Mutual aid* refers to a process whereby members help one another through sharing, problem solving, and support (Gitterman & Shulman, 1994; Steinberg, 2004). In discussing mutual aid in adolescent groups, Malekoff (2004) highlighted the relationships among the members. Group treatment offers students the chance to experience mutual support from peers and to feel that others are "in the same boat" (Mishna & Muskat, 2004a). According to interpersonal group theory, the prime therapeutic factor occurs through interactions in the here-and-now (Yalom & Lescz, 2005). The opportunity to interact with peers and receive feedback in a supportive context fosters cognitive and emotional learning.

The group was also guided by ecological theory. An ecological approach has an emphasis on the larger context and multiple factors that affect a student, rather than a focus mainly on deficits of the child and family (Brown, D'Emidio-Cason, & Benard, 2001). Morrison and Cosden (1997) use the term *ecocultural fit* to describe the relationship between individuals and their environments, including the meaning of an LD for individuals, families, and cultures. School climate encompasses the attitudes, values, and norms that sanction how a school operates (McEvoy & Welker, 2000). The effect of an LD may be compounded by stigma and misconceptions and by an unresponsive school system (Baker & Donelly, 2001).

Pilot Manualization of the Group

The group approach used in the project builds upon previous research conducted by the authors. As this group was part of a larger study, a manual was developed to explicate and evaluate the model. The manual was created in partnership with a children's mental health agency specializing in the mental health needs of children and youth with LD (Muskat, 2004). Thus, the manual was informed by the expertise of social workers who have many years of experience leading groups for students with LD.

Development of group approach. The group model piloted in the current study has undergone a developmental process involving ongoing revision, within a community agency serving children and adolescents with LD (Mishna, Kaiman, Little, & Tarshis, 1994; Mishna, 1996a, b; Mishna & Muskat, 1998, 2001, 2004a, b; Mishna, Muskat, & Schamess, 2002). Initial support for this approach was demonstrated in a qualitative study (Mishna, 1996a, b) and in the aforementioned school-based intervention for students with LD (Mishna & Muskat, 2004a). The current group model includes modifications that incorporate information from the findings of the research previously conducted by the authors, on this particular group approach, together with research evidence on LD and on group work. In addition, the current model is informed by practice wisdom regarding relevant issues that affect students with LD.

There are well-documented advantages and critiques of treatment manuals (see Carroll & Nuro, 2002; Galinsky et al., 2006; McMurran & Duggan, 2005, for detailed discussion). Advantages include having a description of the rationale and procedures as well as detailed session plans. Because manualization enhances treatment integrity, it is considered crucial for evaluation and replication (McMurran & Duggan, 2005). Critiques include the view that these models can be prescriptive and therefore not tailored for diverse populations, and the decreased focus on the treatment alliance or member interaction (Carroll & Nuro, 2002; Chopita, 2002; Kurland & Salmon, 2002; Westen, Novotny, & Thompson-Brenner, 2004). Moreover, manualized treatments are considered to be driven in part by managed care in the United States and by the need to "do more with less" due to decreased government funding for children's treatment in Canada and the United States (Carroll & Nuro, 2002; Kurland & Salmon, 2002).

Group Description

As previously stated, the group utilized self-psychology, mutual aid, and interpersonal group treatment. The topic of LD was woven into discussions. Leaders used techniques to accommodate the LD and foster the group process (Mishna, 1996a, b). The groups also included explicit instructions to increase the members' understanding of LD and to develop their self-advocacy skills. The content included material and discussion related to LD, strengths and coping mechanisms, and activities and role-plays to help group members apply and integrate the content and to enjoy themselves.

An emphasis was placed on helping the members to understand their academic strengths and obtain assistance from teachers, parents, and peers. In addition, attention was paid to bullying, as this population is vulnerable to be bullied (Mishna, 2003; Thompson, Whitney, & Smith, 1994). Materials developed by the researchers and completed by the members throughout the group were placed in folders, which were given to members at the end of the group. The ending was marked by a review of learning and a party/award ceremony.

The groups were co-led by agency and school board social workers and psychologists. Prior to the intervention, agency staff provided school board staff training on group treatment for students with LD and on this manualized approach. Eight groups were held over the 2 years of the larger project. The groups were held weekly for students with LD in Grades 6 through 8, with five to eight members in each group. The groups were held at school, during the school day with attempts to minimize the amount of time students missed class. Group sessions were 12 weeks long for 60 minutes. The literature supports this length for school-based groups (Brown et al., 2001). After each session, leaders completed a checklist to assess treatment fidelity.

EVALUATION

The goals of the group were to increase students' understanding of their LD, increase their self-advocacy skills, improve their adjustment and self-concept, and decrease loneliness. Another goal was to conduct a pilot evaluation of the manualized group treatment for students with LD.

The original sample that participated in the overall school-based research intervention comprised 68 students. Eighteen withdrew at some point before completion of the research project (14 no longer wished to participate and 4 moved), leaving a final sample of 50.

Selected children in the group treatment were invited to take part in individual interviews to obtain their views of the group and the overall research and of such issues as perceived social support. An interview guide was developed by the research team in consultation with the school and agency staff. Purposive sampling was utilized with respect to such variables as gender, grade, nature of difficulty, and school attended to obtain a wide as possible range of experiences (Lincoln & Guba, 1985). Interviews were conducted with 14 students and their parents and teachers. One parent agreed to participate but did not return calls, and thus there were a total of 41 interviews, at which point there was category saturation (McCracken, 1988). Each student and teacher interview took place at the schools and lasted approximately 1 hour; parent interviews were conducted over the phone. Interviews were recorded and transcribed. Several measures were taken to ensure trustworthiness (Lincoln, 1995; Lincoln & Guba, 1985). The researchers' prolonged engagement through many years of practice and research with children who have LD helped to build trust. Triangulation was achieved through the multiple perspectives obtained by interviewing the children, their parents, and teachers. Nvivo software was used to help organize the data (Richards, 1999). Presenting respondents' developing themes addressed member checking. The data were analyzed through constant comparison to develop groupings of similar concepts of participants' perspectives (Creswell, 1998). Consistent and contradictory themes were identified and compared within and across groups of participants. The study received approval from the University of Toronto Research Ethics Board and the school board.

Preliminary Findings: Interviews with Children, Teachers, and Parents

We have tentative results based on preliminary analysis of the individual interviews with the students, teachers, and parents on their views of the group intervention.

Preliminary Data Analysis

Qualitative analytical methods were utilized to draw from the depth and richness of the data. Interviews were assessed in groups by interview subject, with analysis completed separately for students, teachers, and parents using the data-driven inductive approach (Boyatzis, 1998). After reviewing the interviews, the researchers moved to describing and classifying the data according to broad categories (Creswell, 1998) that encompassed the positive and negative group experiences, the experience of the group process, and the child's LD. Inductive data analysis was conducted using a constant comparative method, a technique from grounded theory (Glaser & Strauss, 1967). Negative cases were noted and included in the preliminary analysis. This process was replicated for each group of interviewees—students, parents, and teachers.

Students. It emerged that very few students "chose" to attend the group, and students explained that their parents or teachers "made the decision." However, most indicated that they were pleased to attend once they started. One student reported thanking his parents for "putting me in the group." The students all stated that participating in the group was beneficial and recommended that the group continue to be offered to other students. When referring to the group, a female respondent said "sometimes they can really bring up your spirits." When asked what was most helpful in group, one student responded by stating, "how to pinpoint your disability, and I liked the food." Another participant explained, "And I liked it because it calms me down, like when we talk about our anger. We talk about, like before I used to be scared that I have a learning disability. Now I don't care because I can tell anybody." Differences of opinion regarding the group emerged. For instance, one student wished he could attend the whole group again, whereas another depicted the group as "boring" and "annoying." When asked about ways in which the group was not helpful, still another commented, "Like I think that some parts of it, like I wouldn't use them, but just like bits by bits of information, like I learned something that I wouldn't use and that I would."

Most of the students preferred to have the group occur in school, as this was convenient; one student commented that he would have preferred to attend the group in a different location. The main concern students identified about the group taking place in their schools was being called over the loudspeaker to attend. Some students disliked fielding questions from other students about where they were going, as evident by the following quotation by a participant: "The only reason I didn't like it and then kids are always like, 'Why are you going downstairs?' One kid actually asked me right now, today, before I came down." In contrast, a number of the students stated that their friends knew they attended the group and that it was "not a big deal."

The students all expressed feeling understood by the group leaders. They enjoyed the activities, in particular those that were dissimilar to school, and they especially enjoyed the snacks. Few reported that they talked to anyone about the group. Despite the students' sense that the group was beneficial, many were unsure whether their parents or teachers perceived improvements. However, a number were certain their parents and teachers would notice such changes as their increased confidence and knowledge of their LD. For instance, one participant stated that his parents "really liked me going to the group because before that they really wanted me to learn about how come I had the disability and that. And when there was no programs that would tell me that before and my parents felt really good when I went to the group."

With the majority self-identifying as having an LD (11), the students reported that they learned about their LD and how it influenced their school-work as well as other areas of their lives. The students stated that the group helped them to believe that an LD did not mean they were "dumb," and did not mean they should feel badly about themselves. This recognition was particularly focused on being able to tell others about their LD and to ask questions in class, as the following quotation illustrates: "I was working on a question where no matter what I did, I could not get it and I was just getting frustrated. So I finally worked up enough courage to go, and asked." This ability represented a significant change for the student, who reported that in response, the teacher "helped."

The students reported learning that asking for help was not equated with lacking intelligence. Most attributed their greater ability to ask questions to their participation in the group, and all provided at least one example whereby they received help after having asked a question. Many credited a group simulation exercise in which members role-played asking for help. One student depicted the group as helping him change from being "scared to tell people I have a learning disability" to being able to talk about it without trepidation. Another participant explained, "well like you could feel really down about having a learning disability and they would make you feel, like it's okay, you can't help it, you were just born with it. You can't change it." Another participant noticed a change with respect to how other students responded, saying that in comparison to the year before, "they don't make fun of me no more. They try to understand my learning disability."

Other benefits of group that the students identified included feeling calmer and dealing better with anger, feeling less afraid of telling others they had an LD, and having greater self-awareness and ability to support their friends who have LD. A number of students disclosed that they were bullied because of their LD and that as a result had come to believe the labels they were called, such as "stupid." As one student poignantly articulated, other students, "said I was stupid, that 'you go to the stupid class.'" When asked what it was like having a LD, this participant explained, "I kind of don't like it and I kind of do because the work is easier, but also it's like everybody thinks I'm stupid, but they don't understand what a learning disability is. A learning disability is like you have a higher IQ, but you learn differently." In response to being called names by peers due to the LD, the participant reported, "well, when they call me stupid I think I'm stupid too, sometimes."

The students reported that the group helped them to be able to walk away and tell a teacher when they were bullied. They also talked about the importance of standing up for other students who were bullied. As one participant explained, "I learned to keep, like how to if someone is bullying, like just to walk away when somebody bullies me." Another stated that as a result of the group, "now I know how to talk to people and if I get bullied I know what to say," and still another participant asserted that through the group, "it tells you like how to stop bullying and all that … don't bully others. Don't be a bully. Stick up for people who are being bullied."

Several students were profoundly affected by finding out that successful individuals, such as celebrities, had an LD. As one surprised student exclaimed, "I didn't think famous people could get learning disabilities." This information helped them to believe that an LD need not prevent them from becoming successful. For example one student explained, "well they're famous and he has a learning disability, so anything can happen."

Very few students reported having talked to their parents, teachers, or friends about having an LD. They were especially reluctant to talk to friends about their LD and intensely disliked classroom activities that highlighted their LD, such as reading aloud. There were some differences, for instance, some students identified benefits of LD, such as having a smaller amount and easier school work. The students varied in their views of the public perception of LD. Some believed that people generally viewed individuals with LD as "lazy" and "stupid," whereas others thought individuals with LD were considered "smarter," or "just different." Many students felt their teachers should learn more about LD and be more patient, and several reported teachers "yelling" at them because they did not understand a concept or question, as illustrated by the following quotation: "Just like last month I think, I remember this part that I didn't get this thing on my math and I was asking the teacher and she started to get frustrated and started yelling at me and then she said 'how do you not get it' and stuff like that, in front of everybody too, so I hate it when teachers do that." One participant recommended, "maybe my teachers, they're supposed to go to this learning disability thing that the learning disability teachers go to and they learn a whole bunch of stuff and then they don't get frustrated so easily."

Teachers. The teachers varied in their assessment of the group's benefits. Some did not identify change in the students, whereas others noted benefits for the students such as increased confidence and awareness of their LD, and greater ability to complete school work, attend and participate in class, advocate for their learning needs, and tell teachers when they were bullied. One teacher stated, "As a result of the group, [child] has become more his own self-advocate," and another teacher maintained that "this program allows [child] to speak and say what he feels and talk to others about how he feels." One teacher noticed less conflict involving students who participated in the group along with greater class participation. As a teacher commented, "[child] is really involved in everything that he always wanted to be involved." Still another teacher felt the project benefited the entire school in that it "gives students with learning disabilities a voice in the school." Some teachers expressed concerns about the group, such as students missing class. A few teachers echoed the students' statement that a focus of the intervention should be working with teachers.

Parents. The students' parents identified several benefits they believed were associated with the group. Some benefits were related to school work, such as an increase in motivation and ability of the students to concentrate and learn. With respect to other areas, parents believed the group helped their children to be calmer and to have greater self-esteem and confidence in undertaking tasks and asking for help. A parent commented that as a result of the group their child gained awareness of their strengths, weaknesses, and areas with which they needed help. Another parent noted that "the kids in the group developed more respect for each other at the end of the day." One parent stated that because of the group, "[child] said to me that he doesn't feel lost anymore." Still another reported that her son exclaimed one day after the group, "I'm not lazy! Today in the group I found out I'm not lazy; it's just that I learn differently. I can be a somebody and go to university." Some parents felt the group should be expanded to all grades, and others thought it should be offered over a longer time period. Similar to the teachers, a few parents stated that they would have liked to receive more updates regarding their child's progress, and some expressed concern about their child missing class to attend the group.

PRELIMINARY FINDINGS: MANUAL

The group leaders initially expressed skepticism about using the manual, primarily out of a concern that it would be prescriptive and therefore inhibit leader and member interaction and spontaneity. However, the leaders reported that over time they gained comfort using the manual. They were able to cover all of the content, although some leaders reported changing the timing of some material to meet group needs. For example, members in one group raised the issue of bullying in a session earlier than its sequence in the manual. The leaders conferred and modified that week to cover the topic of bullying in that session, as they did not want to "miss the moment." However, they made sure to discuss material from that week's content in the following session. A number of group leaders added activities that they felt better addressed the content that was to be covered. In all cases, they recorded the changes and the new content.

PRACTICE PRINCIPLES

This article reports on the perceptions of middle-school students with LD, their parents and teachers regarding the children's participation in a school-based group with the aims of increasing the students' knowledge and understanding of LD and of their own learning strengths and deficits, and increasing their ability to advocate for themselves. Preliminary findings of the interviews with selected students who participated in the group, and their parents and teachers suggest that the group was beneficial in ways that ameliorated risk factors and promoted protective factors identified in the literature. The group was identified by the children and their parents and teachers as improving the students' knowledge of LD and of their own particular learning strengths and difficulties and as increasing their ability to assert themselves and ask for help.

Based on the preliminary analysis of the interviews, tentative recommendations for practice have been identified, which parallel protective factors identified in the literature. The following practice principles are offered as guidelines.

1. Increase teachers' and parents' understanding of LD: For students to understand and cope with their LD, they require the assistance of those closest to them. Misinformation about LD that children and youth with LD receive from parents and teachers can have negative and painful consequences for students (Higgins, Raskind, Goldberg, & Herman, 2002). There have been many calls for better teacher training to help them understand LD and develop practices that effectively address the LD

(Hehir, 2002). Parents and teachers must have accurate and current information and knowledge about LD so they can truly support students to succeed academically and socially.

2. Group workers must meet with parents and if possible, with teachers: The teachers and parents expressed their desire to be provided with more regular information regarding the group content and student progress. It is well established that the support and assistance of family, teachers, and other helping professionals are crucial for individuals with LD to succeed as adults (Barga, 1996; Gerber, Ginsberg, & Reiff, 1992). An ecological approach to intervention supports the principle of communication among the many contexts in which the student interacts. Creation of a support team for students struggling with LD comprised of the student and his or her teachers and parents can help the student develop, practice, and consolidate self-advocacy skills, so critical for their future endeavours.

3. Foster communication between parents and teachers with students about their LD: Similar to the findings in the literature (Eisenman & Tascione, 2002), the students in the current study reported that their parents or teachers rarely spoke with them about their LD. Although a number of the students stated that they did not initially wish to attend the group and that the parts of the group they enjoyed the most were activities that were unlike school, for the most part the students stated that learning about LD in general and their own LD in particular was helpful. Moreover, most of the students were able to provide examples that indicated how this information benefited them. This finding lends support to the need for discussion about LD with the students themselves to enhance their ability to assert their needs, despite the difficulties associated with this process (Eisenman & Tascione, 2002; Merchant & Gajar, 1997). Thus, it is incumbent upon social workers and other school-based practitioners to work with parents and teachers in helping them find developmentally appropriate ways to discuss LD in general and children's specific LD.

4. Ensure that the issue of bullying is investigated and addressed: Based on the research to date, there is reason to believe that children with LD are at greater risk for victimization (Thompson et al., 1994; Whitney, Nabuzoka, & Smith, 1992). Corresponding with these findings, many of the students in the current study reported that they were bullied, which was addressed in the group. A few of the students stated that they believed their participation in the group allowed them to tell a teacher about their bullying experiences. This finding is very important because teachers and parents are often unaware that a child has been bullied because many children do not admit to being victimized (Casey-Cannon, Hayward, & Gowe, 2001; Mishna, 2004; Pepler, Craig, Ziegler, & Charach, 1994). Despite their reluctance to report bullying, victimized children who do tell often find interventions by their parents, teachers, and peers effective (Smith & Shu, 2000), which "reinforces the importance of breaking the 'culture of silence'" (Smith & Shu, 2000, p. 210).

5. In school-based interventions, be sensitive to the stigma associated with LD: Despite the many benefits of offering group in schools, one risk is increasing a child's negative experiences such as bullying or feelings of shame due to the associated stigma. A few students in the current study noted the bullying they endured as a result of leaving class to attend the group as one disadvantage of holding the group in the school. Therefore, group workers must collaborate closely with teachers and school administrators and involve the students in determining unobtrusive ways through which the students can attend group.

6. Ensure that manuals are used flexibly and address the needs of a particular group: It is well documented that treatment manuals provide a framework to deliver a specific practice approach and offer strategies to achieve the purpose of the intervention. However, there is growing awareness of the need to adapt the approach and manual to the needs of the particular clients (Galinsky et al., 2006; Kendall, Chu, Gifford, Hayes, & Nauta, 1998). The group leaders in the current study stressed the need for flexibility in offering the group, and, according to preliminary analysis, such flexibility was essential to the effective delivery of the groups. The use of manualized approaches in group work requires integrating the content of the manualized program with sound approaches to group leadership and understanding of group dynamics. In particular, practitioners are encouraged to use their creativity in order to bring manuals to life.

CONCLUSION

We have described a pilot of a manualized group intervention, which was one component of a larger collaborative school-based intervention for middle-school students with LD. We hope the results of the comprehensive evaluation will offer guidance in the creation of future school-based interventions for students with LD. Any practice intervention such as this school-based program cannot be truly evaluated without examining the challenges that arise (Nastasi & Schensul, 2005). Accordingly, we will systematically document and examine challenges as well as factors that promote the intervention.

ACKNOWLEDGMENT

This study was funded by a grant from the Social Sciences and Humanities Research Council of Canada. We acknowledge the support of the Toronto Catholic District School Board psychologists, social workers, teachers, and administrators, and the children and their parents, in particular Maria Kokai. We would like to thank Integra group leaders and administration, research assistants, and especially the research project coordinator Arija Birze.

REFERENCES

Akos, P. (2000). Building empathic skills in elementary school children through group work. *Journal for Specialists in Group Work, 25*(2), 214–223.

Al-Yagon, M., & Mikulincer, M. (2004). Patterns of close relationships and socioemotional and academic adjustment among school-age children with learning disabilities. *Learning Disabilities Research & Practice, 19*(1), 12–19.

Baker, K., & Donelly, M. (2001). The social experiences of children with disability and the influence of environment: A framework for intervention. *Disability and Society, 16*(1), 71–85.

Barga, N. K. (1996). Students with learning disabilities in education: Managing a disability. *Journal of Learning Disabilities, 29*(4), 413–421.

Berg, R. C., & Wages, L. (1982). Group counseling with the adolescent learning disabled. *Journal of Learning Disabilities, 15*(5), 276–277.

Berkovitz, I. H. (1989). Application of group therapy in secondary schools. In F. J. C. Azima & L. H. Richmond (Eds.), *Adolescent group psychotherapy* (pp. 99–123). Madison, WI: International Universities Press, Inc.

Boyatzis, R. (1998). *Transforming qualitative information: Thematic analysis and code development*. Thousand Oaks, CA: Sage.

Bratton, S. C., Ray, D., Rhine, T., & Jones, L. (2005). The efficacy of play therapy with children: A meta-analytic review of treatment outcomes. *Professional Psychology: Research and Practice, 36*(4), 376–390.

Bronfenbrenner, U. (1986). Ecology of the family as a context for human development: Research perspectives. *Developmental Psychology, 22*(6), 723–742.

Bronfenbrenner, U. (1994). Ecological models of human development. In T. Husén & T. N. Postlethwaite (Eds.), *The international encyclopedia of education* (2nd ed., Vol. 3, pp. 1643–1647). Oxford, UK: Pergamon Press.

Brown, J. H., D'Emidio-Cason, M., & Benard, B. (2001). *Resilience education*. Thousand Oaks, CA: Corwin Press.

Carabine, B., & Downton, R. (2000). Specific learning disabilities and peer support. *Educational Psychology in Practice, 16*, 487–494.

Carroll, K. M., & Nuro, K. M. (2002). One size cannot fit all: A stage model for psychotherapy manual development. *Clinical Psychology: Science and Practice, 9*(4), 396–406.

Casey-Cannon, S., Hayward, C., & Gowen, K. (2001) Middle-school girls' reports of peer victimization: Concerns, consequences, and implications. *Professional School Counseling, 5*(2), 138–153.

Chopita, B. F. (2002) Treatment manuals for the real world: Where do we build them? *Clinical Psychology: Science and Practice, 9*(4), 431–433.

Cosden, M. (2001). Risk and resilience for substance abuse among adolescents and adults with LD. *Journal of Learning Disabilities, 34*(4), 352–358.

Cosden, M., Brown, C., & Elliott, K. (2002). Development of self-understanding and self -esteem in children and adults with learning disabilities. In B. Y. L. Wong, & M. L. Donahue (Eds.), *The social dimensions of learning disabilities: Essays in honor of Tanis Bryan* (pp. 33–51). Mahwah, NJ: Lawrence Erlbaum.

Cramer-Azima, F. J. (2002). Group psychotherapy for children and adolescents. In M. Lewis (Ed.), *Child and adolescent psychiatry: A comprehensive textbook* (3rd ed., pp. 1032–1036). Philadelphia: Lippincott, Williams & Wilkins.

Creswell, J. (1998). *Qualitative inquiry and research design: Choosing among five traditions.*Thousand Oaks, CA: Sage.

DeLucia-Waack, J. L. (2000). Effective group work in the schools. *Journal for Specialists in Group Work, 25*(2), 131–132.

Dishion, T. J., & Kavanagh, K. (2000). A multilevel approach to family-centered prevention in schools: Process and outcome. *Addictive Behaviors, 25*(6), 899–911.

Eisenman, L. T., & Tascione, L. (2002). "How come nobody told me?" Fostering self realization through a high-school English curriculum. *Learning Disabilities Research & Practice, 17*(1), 35–46.

Elbaum, B., & Vaughn, S. (2001). School-based interventions to enhance the self-concept of students with learning disabilities: A meta-analysis. *The Elementary School Journal, 101*(3), 303–329.

Farrell, A. D., Meyer, A. L., & Dahlberg, L. L. (1996). Richmond youth against violence: A school-based program for urban adolescents. *American Journal of Preventive Medicine, 12*(5, Suppl), 13–21.

Freeman, J. G., Stoch, S. A., Chan, J. S. N., & Hutchinson, N. L. (2004). Academic resilience: A retrospective study of adults with learning difficulties. *Alberta Journal of Educational Research, 50*(1), 5–21.

Galinsky, M., Terzian, M. A., & Fraser, M. (2006). The art of group work practice with manualized curricula. *Social Work with Groups, 29*(1), 11–26.

Gerber, P. J., Ginsberg, R., & Reiff, H. B. (1992). Identifying alterable patterns in employment success for highly successful adults with learning disabilities. *Journal of Learning Disabilities, 25*(8), 475–487.

Germain, C. B., & Bloom, M. (1999). *Human behavior in the social environment: An ecological view* (2nd ed.). New York: Columbia University Press.

Gitterman, A., & Shulman, L. (1994). *Mutual aid groups, vulnerable populations and the life cycle.* New York: Columbia University Press.

Glaser, B., & Strauss, A. (1967). *The discovery of grounded theory: Strategies of qualitative research.* London: Wiedenfeld and Nicholson.

Greenham, S. (1999). Learning disabilities and psychosocial adjustment: A critical review. *Child Neuropsychology, 5*, 171–196.

Gresham, F. M., Sugai, G., & Horner, R. H. (2001). Interpreting outcomes of social skills training for students with high-incidence disabilities. *Exceptional Children, 67*(3), 331–344.

Hehir, T. (2002). Eliminating ableism in education. *Harvard Educational Review, 72* (1), 1–32.

Higgins, E. L., Raskind, M. H., Goldberg, R. J., & Herman, K. L. (2002). Stages of acceptance of a learning disability: The impact of labeling. *Learning Disability Quarterly, 25*(1), 3–18.

Hoag, M. J., & Burlingame, G. M. (1997). Child and adolescent group psychotherapy: A narrative review of effectiveness and the case for meta-analysis. *Journal of Child and Adolescent Group Therapy, 7*(2), 51–68.

Kendall, P. C., Chu, B., Gifford, A., Hayes, C., & Nauta, M. (1998). Breathing life into a manual: Flexibility and creativity with manual-based treatments. *Cognitive and Behavioral Practice, 5*, 177–198.

Kohut, H. (1984). *How does analysis cure?* Chicago & London: University of Chicago Press.

Kuperminc, G. P., Leadbeater, B. J., & Blatt, S. J. (2001). School social climate and individual differences in vulnerability to psychopathology among middle school students. *Journal of School Psychology, 39*(2), 141–159.

Kurland, R., & Salmon, R. (2002). *Caught in the doorway between education and practice: Group work's battle for survival*. Plenary Address, 24th Annual Symposium of the Association of the Advancement of Social Work with Groups, Brooklyn, N.Y.

Lincoln, Y. S. (1995). Emerging criteria for quality in qualitative and interpretive research. *Qualitative Inquiry, 1*(3), 275–289.

Lincoln, Y. S., & Guba, E. (1985). *Naturalistic inquiry*. Beverly Hills, CA: Sage.

Lomonaco, S., Scheidlinger, S., & Aronson, S. (2000). Five decades of children's group treatment—An overview. *Journal of Child and Adolescent Group Therapy, 10,* 77–96.

Maag, J. W., & Reid, R. (2006). Depression among students with learning disabilities: Assessing the risk. *Journal of Learning Disabilities, 39*(1), 3–10.

Malekoff, A. (2004). *Group work with adolescents: Principles and practice, second edition*. New York: Guilford Press.

Margalit, M. (2004). Second-generation research on resilience: Social-emotional aspects of children with learning disabilities. *Learning Disabilities Research & Practice, 19*(1), 45–48.

Margalit, M., & Al-Yagon, M. (2002). The loneliness experience of children with learning disabilities. In B. Wong & M. Donahue (Eds.), *The social dimensions of learning disabilities: Essays in honor of Tanis Bryan* (pp. 53–75). Mahwah, NJ: Lawrence Erlbaum.

Mason, C., Field, S., & Sawilowsky, S. (2004). Implementation of self-determination activities and student participation in IEP's. *Exceptional Children, 70*(4), 441–451.

McEvoy, A., & Welker, R. (2000). Antisocial behaviour, academic failure, and school climate: A critical review. *Journal of Emotional and Behavioral Disorders, 8*(3), 130–140.

McIntosh, R., & Vaughn, S. (1993). So you want to teach social skills to your students: Some pointers from the research. *Exceptionality Education Canada, 3*(1/2), 39–59.

McCracken, G. (1988). *The long interview*. Thousand Oaks, CA: Sage.

McMurran, M., & Duggan, C. (2005). The manualization of a treatment programme for personality disorder. *Criminal Behaviour and Mental Health, 15,* 17–27.

McNamara, J. K., Willoughby, T., Chalmers, H., & YLC-CURA . (2005). Psychosocial status of adolescents with learning disabilities with and without comorbid attention deficit disorder. *Learning Disabilities Research & Practice, 20*(4), 234–244.

Merchant, D. J., & Gajar, A. (1997). A review of the literature on self advocacy components in transition programs for students with learning disabilities. *Journal of Vocational Rehabilitation, 8,* 223–231.

Meyer, A. L., & Farrell, A. D. (1998). Social skills training to promote resilience in urban sixth-grade students: One product of an action research strategy to prevent youth violence in high-risk environments. *Education and Treatment of Children, 21*(4), 461–488.

Miller, M. (2002). Resilience elements in students with learning disabilities. *Journal of Clinical Psychology: A Second Generation of Resilience Research, 58*(3), 291–298.

Mishna, F. (1996a). Finding their voice: Group therapy for adolescents with learning disabilities. *Learning Disabilities, Research & Practice, 11*, 249–258.

Mishna, F. (1996b). In their own words: Therapeutic factors for adolescents who have learning disabilities. *International Journal of Group Psychotherapy, 46*, 265–273.

Mishna, F. (2003). Learning disabilities and bullying: Double jeopardy. *Journal of Learning Disabilities, 36*(4), 336–347.

Mishna, F. (2004). A qualitative study of bullying from multiple perspectives. *Children & Schools, 26*(4), 234–247.

Mishna, F., Kaiman, J., Little, S., & Tarshis, E. (1994). Group therapy with adolescents who have learning disabilities and social/emotional problems. *Journal of Child and Adolescent Group Therapy, 4*, 117–131.

Mishna, F., & Muskat, B. (1998). Group therapy for boys with features of Asperger syndrome and concurrent learning disabilities: Finding a peer group. *Journal of Child and Adolescent Group Therapy, 8*(3), 97–114.

Mishna, F., & Muskat, B. (2001). Social group work for young offenders with learning disabilities. *Social Work with Groups, 24*(3/4), 11–31.

Mishna, F., & Muskat, B. (2004a). "I'm not the only one!" Group therapy for children and adolescents with learning disabilities. *International Journal of Group Psychotherapy, 54*(4), 455–476.

Mishna, F., & Muskat, B. (2004b). School-based group treatment for students with learning disabilities: A collaborative approach. *Children & Schools, 26*(3), 135–150.

Mishna, F., Muskat, B., & Schamess, G. (2002). Food for thought: The use of food in group therapy with children and adolescents. *International Journal of Group Psychotherapy, 52*(1), 27–47.

Morrison, G., & Cosden, M. (1997). Risk, resilience and adjustment of individuals with learning disabilities. *Learning Disability Quarterly, 20*(1), 43–60.

Muskat, B. (2004). *Project inside and out: Enhancing self understanding in students with learning disabilities group work manual.* Unpublished manual. Integra Foundation.

Nabuzoka, D. (2003). Teacher ratings and peer nominations of bullying and other behaviour of children with and without learning difficulties. *Educational Psychology, 23*, 307–321.

Nastasi, B. K., & Schensul, S. L. (2005). Contributions of qualitative research to the validity of intervention research. *Journal of School Psychology, 43*(3), 177–195.

Offord, D. R., Boyle, M., & Racine, Y. (1990). *Ontario child health study: Children at risk.* Ontario, Canada: Ministry of Community and Social Services.

Page, R. C., Weiss, J. F., & Lietaer, G. (2001). Humanistic group psychotherapy. In D. J. Cain & J. Seeman (Eds.), *Humanistic psychotherapies: Handbook of research and practice* (pp. 339–368). Washington, DC: American Psychological Association.

Palmer, S. B., & Wehmeyer, M. L. (2003). Promoting self-determination in early elementary school: Teaching self-regulated problem-solving and goal-setting skills. *Remedial and Special Education, 24*(2), 115–126.

Pavri, S., & Hegwer-DiVita, M. (2006). Meeting the social and emotional needs of students with disabilities: The special educators' perspective. *Reading & Writing Quarterly, 22*(2), 139–153.

Pearl, R., & Bay, M. (1999). Psychosocial correlates of learning disabilities. In V. L. Schwean & D. H. Saklofske (Eds.), *Handbook of psychosocial characteristics of exceptional children* (pp. 443–470). New York: Kluwer Academic/ Plenum Publishers.

Pepler, D. J., Craig, W. M., Ziegler, S., & Charach, A. (1994). An evaluation of an anti-bullying intervention in Toronto schools. *Canadian Journal of Community Mental Health, 13*(2), 95–110.

Pollio, D. E. (2002). The evidence-based group worker. *Social Work with Groups, 25*(4), 57–70.

Raskind, M. H., Goldberg, R. J., Higgins, E. L., & Herman, K. L. (1999). Patterns of change and predictors of success in individuals with learning disabilities: Results from a twenty-year longitudinal study. *Learning Disabilities Research and Practice, 14*, 35–49.

Richards, L. (1999). *Using Nvivo in qualitative research.* Bundoora, Australia: Qualitative Solutions and Research Pty. Ltd.

Scheidlinger, S., & Aronson, S. (1991). Group psychotherapy of adolescents. In M. Slomowitz (Ed.), *Adolescent psychotherapy* (pp. 101–119). Washington, DC: American Psychiatric Press.

Shechtman, Z., & Pastor, R. (2005). Cognitive-behavioral and humanistic group treatment for children with learning disabilities: A comparison of outcomes and process. *Journal of Counseling Psychology, 52*(3), 322–336.

Simons-Morton, B. G., Crump, A. D., Haynie, D. L., & Saylor, K. E. (1999). Student-school bonding and adolescent problem behavior. *Health Education Research, 14*(1), 99–107.

Sinclair, M. F., Christenson, S. L., Evelo, D. L., & Hurley, C. M. (1998). Dropout prevention for youth with disabilities: Efficacy of a sustained school engagement procedure. *Exceptional Children, 65*(1), 7–21.

Smith, P. K., & Shu, S. (2000). What good school can do about bullying: Findings from a survey in English schools after a decade of research and action. *Childhood, 7*(2), 193–212.

Sorensen, L. G., Forbes, P. W., Bernstein, J. H., Weiler, M. D., Mitchell, W. M., & Waber, D. P. (2003). Psychosocial adjustment over a two year period in children referred for learning problems: Risk, resilience, and adaptation. *Learning Disabilities Research and Practice, 18*(1), 10–24.

Steinberg, D. M. (2004). *The mutual-aid approach to working with groups: Helping people help one another.* New York: Haworth Press.

Stone, C. A., & May, A. L. (2002). The accuracy of academic self-evaluations in adolescents with learning disabilities. *Journal of Learning Disabilities, 35*(4), 370–383.

Svetaz, M. V., Ireland, M., & Blum, R. (2000). Adolescents with learning disabilities: Risk and protective factors associated with emotional well-being: Findings from the National Longitudinal Study of Adolescent Health. *Journal of Adolescent Health, 27*, 340–348.

Thompson, D., Whitney, I., & Smith, I. (1994). Bullying of children with special needs in mainstream schools. *Support for Learning, 9*(3), 103–106.

Vaughn, S., Elbaum, B., & Boardman, A. G. (2001). The social functioning of students with learning disabilities: Implications for inclusion. *Exceptionality*, *9*(1/2), 47–65.

Wehmeyer, M. L., Field, S., Doren, B., Jones, B., & Mason, C. (2004).Self-determination and students' involvement in standards-based reform. *Exceptional Children*, *70*(4), 413–425.

Weist, M. D., Nabors, L. A., Myers, C. P., & Armbruster, P. (2000). Evaluation of expanded school mental health programs. *Community Mental Health Journal*, *36*(4), 395–411.

Weisz, J. R., Weiss, B., Han, S. S., Granger, D. A., & Morton, T. (1995). Effects of psychotherapy with children and adolescents revisited: A meta-analysis of treatment outcome studies. *Psychological Bulletin*, *117*, 450–468.

Westen, D., Novotny, C. M., & Thompson-Brenner, H. (2004). The empirical status of empirically supported psychotherapies: Assumptions, findings, and reporting in controlled clinical trials. *Psychological Bulletin*, *130*(4), 631–663.

Whitney, I., Nabuzoka, D., & Smith, P. K. (1992). Bullying in schools: Mainstream and special needs. *Support for Learning*, *7*(1), 3–7.

Wiener, J. (2002). Friendship and social adjustment of children with learning disabilities. In B. Wong, & M. Donahue (Eds.), *The social dimensions of learning disabilities: Essays in honor of Tanis Bryan* (pp. 93–114). Mahwah, NJ: Lawrence Erlbaum.

Wiener, J. (2003). Resilience and multiple risks: A response to Bernice Wong. *Learning Disabilities Research & Practice*, *18*(2), 77–81.

Yalom, I. D., & Lescz, M. (2005). *The theory and practice of group psychotherapy* (5th ed.). New York: Basic Books.

Releasing the Steam: An Evaluation of the Supporting Tempers, Emotions, and Anger Management (STEAM) Program for Elementary and Adolescent-Age Children

BRUCE A. BIDGOOD

University of Northern British Columbia, Terrace, British Columbia, Canada

HEATHER WILKIE

University of Windsor, Windsor, Ontario, Canada

ANNETTE KATCHALUBA

Kitchener-Waterloo Family & Children's Services, Waterloo, Ontario, Canada

This paper chronicles an evaluation of the Supporting Tempers, Emotions, and Anger Management (STEAM), a school-based emotion management program for elementary and adolescent age children. A quasi-experimental design was used to assess the program impacts as reported by children, their parents, and teachers. The results revealed that STEAM was associated with an array of significant positive changes in both the home and school environment. The program was particularly effective with young children (Grades 1–3) relative to students in the older age cohorts (i.e., Grades 4–6 and 7–8). The findings suggest the importance of early intervention to assist children in the development of emotion management.

Emotions are responses to environmental stimuli that create an intense but short-term affective state. Although they are a natural part of the human experience, many children experience difficulties in managing their emotions in adaptive ways. These difficulties often arise in children because of poor role modeling and a general unawareness that there are positive ways to express and manage emotions (Wilde, 1995). Little data is available on the prevalence of emotional difficulties in children, but rates between 1.2% and 10% have been reported (Achenbach & Elderbrood, 1981; Bower, 1981; Cullinan, Epstein, & Kauffman, 1984; Dice, 1993), with 3 times more males affected than females (Dice, 1993).

Children who are unable to successfully manage their emotions may manifest behavioral difficulties in the home and school environment. This may be disruptive to the classroom and learning atmosphere (Wilde, 1995), and consequently, emotional difficulties have been associated with academic performance (Gumora & Arsenio, 2002) and educational and career outcomes (Eisenberg, Fabes, & Murphy, 1996; Nelson & Colvin, 1996). A child's inability to manage emotions may also lead to poor interpersonal relationships with peers and adults, and future social maladjustment is often predicted for children who are exposed to negative expressions of emotion (Crick, 1996).

Successfully teaching young children about feelings and emotion management increases their ability to understand the feelings of others, their own feelings, and how to appropriately act upon their emotions (Dunn & Brown, 1991; Dupont, 1994). Furthermore, when children are able to control their expression of emotions, they have a higher likelihood of developing prosocial behavior and excelling in interpersonal relationships (Garner & Power, 1996). For these reasons it is important to teach children and adolescents the necessary skills to manage their emotional expressions before any patterns of poor emotional management become ingrained (Osher & Hanley, 1996; Whitesell & Harter, 1996).

Anger is one particular emotion that children often struggle with, and learning to deal with anger has been called one of the "most important maturational tasks of emotional development" (Akande, 1996). A child's inability to properly express anger may lead to internalizing behavior (e.g., depression) and externalizing behavior (e.g., aggression) (Zeman, Shipman, & Suveg, 2002). Research has supported the effectiveness of relaxation strategies and systematic desensitization for use with individuals experiencing problems managing their anger (Ecton & Feindler, 1986). For instance, Zaichkowsky and Zaichkowsky (1984) found that relaxation training reduced the physiological responses of fourth-grade students when exposed to anger-provoking situations. Similar positive results were found when aggressive fourth- and fifth-grade boys received cognitive-behavioral treatment. In this instance, teachers later rated the boys as being less angry and having fewer anger-related problems than those that did not receive treatment (Deffenbacher, Lynch, Oetting, & Kemper, 1996; Sukhodolsky, Solomon, & Perine, 2000).

Although some programs choose to focus exclusively on anger management, programs such as the PATHS (Promoting Alternative Thinking Strategies) curriculum (Greenberg, Kusche, Cook, & Quamma, 1995) focus on the expression, understanding, and regulation of a broader range of emotions. It aims to develop social problem solving through the use of self-control and emotional awareness. Developed for first- to third-grade children, the PATHS curriculum is intended to be taught throughout the school year by regular classroom teachers. PATHS involves the use of such activities as the creation of "Feeling Faces." which allows the children to communicate how they are feeling through the display of various facial expressions. Another activity used in this program is the Control Signals Poster, which uses a stoplight format to walk the child through the necessary steps for social problem solving. Greenberg et al. (1995) demonstrated the effectiveness of this program in regular and special-needs classrooms and reported that PATHS appears to particularly increase children's ability to discuss their feelings and their self-efficacy in controlling their emotional displays.

Some programs such as Second Step (e.g., Frey, Hirschstein, & Guzzo, 2000) combine both approaches by focusing on anger management and generalized emotion management. Second Step, which was first developed in 1986 and has subsequently been used around the globe (Frey et al., 2000), is a primary prevention program to promote social competence through the use of empathy, social problem solving, and anger management. Second Step has lessons that are taught twice a week by regular classroom teachers and has been designed for children from preschool to Grade 9. These program lessons are age appropriate and include such tasks as role-playing, group work, recognizing internal physical cues for anger, stress-reduction techniques, and group discussions (Frey et al., 2000). Research suggests that across all age levels, children who participate in the program display significant increases in social skills knowledge compared to children in control classrooms (e.g., Moore & Beland, 1992). A large-scale behavioral study of 790 second- and third graders also provided evidence that physical aggression was reduced in children randomly assigned to receive this training, relative to children not enrolled in the program (Grossman et al., 1997).

The Supporting Tempers, Emotions, and Anger Management (STEAM) program adopts a similar approach to Second Step by combining generalized emotion management with anger management. It is designed to help children and adolescents by teaching them to identify what emotion they are experiencing and to employ the skills necessary to express their feelings in a positive and healthy manner. The program aims to teach emotion management through an emphasis on self-awareness, triggers of emotions, body signals, and skills to express emotions before the child has lost control. Considerable emphasis is placed on teaching techniques to handle anger, as most students were referred based on their inability to manage this emotion. It was hoped that participation in this program would increase self-control by reducing impulsive behavior, reducing the incidence and intensity of temper situations, strengthening self-esteem, and increasing social support by improving interpersonal skills. The STEAM program is designed to facilitate an interaction between the child's parents and teachers, as research suggests this is the most effective way to produce lasting changes (Friesen & Osher, 1996; Illback & Nelson, 1996; Osher & Hanley, 1996). It was therefore expected that improvements in emotion management would be demonstrated in both the home and school environment.

METHOD

Participants

A total of 143 children participated in the STEAM program. All were recruited from five schools in the Waterloo Region District Separate School Board in Waterloo, Ontario, Canada. The children ranged from Grades 1 to 8, with the following breakdown: Grade 1: $n = 15$; Grade 2: $n = 16$; Grade 3: $n = 35$; Grade 4: $n = 23$; Grade 5: $n = 23$; Grade 6: $n = 13$; Grade 7: $n = 9$; Grade 8: $n = 9$. Although specific demographic information was not collected by the programs to protect the anonymity and confidentiality of participants, anecdotal reports by the leaders revealed that boys and girls were enrolled in each of the groups and that the sample was overwhelmingly White.

Measures

Behavioral and Emotional Rating Scale. The Behavioral and Emotional Rating Scale (BERS; Epstein & Sharma, 1998) is a 52-item questionnaire consisting of statements such as "Identifies own feelings" and "Uses anger management skills." Responses are given on a 0 (*not at all like the child*) to 4 (*very much like the child*) Likert-type scale. These questions assess five dimensions of childhood strengths: Interpersonal Strength, Intrapersonal Strength, School Functioning, Affective Strength, and Family Involvement. The BERS is suitable for use with children ages 5 to 18 and is designed for use by parents and professionals at school or home (Epstein & Sharma, 1998). When administered to children with emotional or behavioral disorders, the BERS has been shown to be reliable and valid. Internal consistency for the five BERS subscales ranges from $\alpha = .84$ to $\alpha = .92$; test–retest reliability ranges from $r = .85$ to $r = .99$; and interrater reliability ranges from $r = .83$ to $r = .96$ (Epstein & Sharma, 1998). The BERS subscales have also been shown to significantly correlate with other measures of social competence and teacher reports (Epstein & Sharma, 1998). The BERS was completed at pre- and posttest by parents and teachers in the current study.

Child self-report. Children were asked to complete an author-compiled 10-item questionnaire assessing their ability to manage their emotions. Items included statements such as, "I can find ways to solve the problems that make me angry" and, "I can tell in my body when my feelings are sneaking in." Responses were given on a 0 (*never*) to 3 (*always*) Likert-type scale. No psychometric information is available for this questionnaire as it was designed specifically for the current study. Children were asked to complete this measure at pre- and posttest.

Procedure

Teachers and school principals were educated regarding the aims of the STEAM program, and these school professionals subsequently referred children that they felt would benefit from involvement. Letters were also sent to parents of all children at each of the participating schools, informing them of the emotions management program and that they could themselves make a referral if they could answer *yes* to any of a series of questions (such as, "Does your child hit or explode if angry?" and "Does your child seem sad or depressed?"). This letter also outlined the timeline of the group meetings and informed them of the opportunity for them to attend parent sessions (including an initial information session on the program). This contact with parents ensured that children who only demonstrated deficits in emotion management within the home environment were also included. All parents gave written consent for their children to participate in the program.

Children who were referred to the STEAM program were then interviewed by a BSW student and were assessed on set criteria, including group readiness, past group experiences, and willingness to participate. Target signs such as low tolerance for frustration, inability to deal with authority figures, and poor self-control were also assessed. Principals, teachers, and group leaders assigned children who were deemed appropriate for the intervention to the group programs until the enrollment capacity was reached. Children who could not immediately be accommodated were assigned to the wait-list and were subsequently offered the program in the following school year.Children were placed into three selected cohorts based on grade: eight Primary groups of Grades 1–3, seven Junior groups of Grades 4–6, and two Intermediate groups of Grades 7–8. Each group consisted of 7 to 11 students. The group format was chosen because this approach has become recognized as the most efficacious form of therapy with children as it normalizes the experiences of children, provides social reinforcement, and assists in the development of interpersonal skills (Rose, 1974; Schiffer, 1984).

The groups met during the normal school day at a local youth center. Children were bussed from their respective schools to the youth center. The STEAM program consisted of 12 sessions, 90 minutes in length, which occurred on a weekly basis. All groups were led by a MSW facilitator and a volunteer co-facilitator (either a MSW, a BSW, or a youth center employee), who received training on this program prior to its initiation.

The STEAM program followed the activity-interview theoretical framework (Schiffer, 1984) by combining play activities with traditional talk therapies techniques, such as group discussion. Activities included such things as relaxation training, role-playing, journaling of the child's feelings, completion of a log of anger-provoking situations, and exercises in self-esteem. These activities were modeled after those used in both the Second Step and PATHS curriculums. Group sessions consisted of an initial emotional check-in (including the use of a temper-a-ture scale), a relaxation exercise, presentation of the material to be covered, a snack, and a closing ritual. Two specific STEAM programs were offered: The Temper Taming Program (for Grades 1 through 6) and the Taming the Dragon Program (for Grades 7 and 8). Both programs covered the same material but differed in activities to ensure that they were age appropriate (see the Appendix for session topics and objectives).

Part of the STEAM program also involved training for school professionals and parents. A designated staff member at each of the participating schools was involved in a $3\frac{1}{2}$-day training session on the concepts of the program. The principal of one of the schools also voluntarily participated in this training. Parents of children in the program were also invited to participate in three voluntary parent-training sessions, held at 6-week intervals throughout the course of the 12-week program. These sessions focused on transferring the skills learned through the STEAM program to the home environment and also allowed the parents to express their experiences of having their child participate in the program. School professionals, group facilitators, and parents were also given a final opportunity to participate in focus groups that discussed the benefits and limitations of the STEAM program.

RESULTS

Teacher Ratings

Teacher-completed BERS were screened, and any questionnaires with more than 10% of the responses missing were excluded. Most excluded questionnaires were missing well over this criterion, and 10% of teacher-completed questionnaires were excluded for the pretest BERS and 5% for the posttest BERS. Remaining questionnaires with missing data were replaced with the mean of that child's score for the particular dimension. Scores for each dimension were calculated as the total of all items comprising each dimension. Due to a large number of missing data (only 35% of children had a complete teacher-reported Family Involvement BERS subscale at pretest), the Family Involvement subscale could not be calculated for the teacher reports.

Although the subscales for each BERS administration were found to be significantly correlated ($p < .001$), the various subscales were analyzed independently in addition to the total score. It was reasoned that analysis at this level would yield useful information and would not obscure potential findings that may not be evident in the total score. It was also felt that analysis of the individual subscales would direct attention to what areas of functioning, if any, were most affected by the STEAM training. No explicit hypotheses regarding differences in the subscales were made.

For students in Grades 1 through 3, teachers reported increases in Interpersonal Strength, $t(49) = -2.52$, $p = .015$; Intrapersonal Strength, $t(49) = -3.82$, $p < .001$; and School Functioning, $t(49) = -2.91$, $p = .005$ (see Table 1). No difference in Affective Strength was found for this group. Analysis of the total BERS scores (based on four subscales) indicated an overall improvement for Grades 1 through 3. Teacher reports revealed no changes on any of the dimensions for Grades 4 through 6 or Grades 7 through 8.

Parent Ratings

Parent-completed BERS were screened in the same manner as those completed by the teachers. This resulted in 7% of completed questionnaires being excluded for the pretest BERS and 1% for the posttest BERS. In contrast to the teachers, all five dimensions could be calculated based on the parent reports. For Grades 1 to 3, parents reported increases in all five dimensions: Interpersonal Strength, $t(35) = -2.50$, $p = .017$; Intrapersonal Strength, $t(35) = -2.38$, $p = .023$; School Functioning, $t(35) = -2.52$, $p = .017$; Affective Strength, $t(35) = -2.51$, $p = .017$; and Family Involvement, $t(35) = -2.19$,

TABLE 1 Teacher Ratings on the Behavioral and Emotional Ratings Scale

	Grades 1–3 ($n = 50$)	Grades 4–6 ($n = 48$)	Grades 7–8 ($n = 13$)
Interpersonal			
Pre	21.58 (9.33)	20.09 (9.26)	18.61 (6.90)
Post	23.74 (9.30)*	20.71 (8.70)	17.47 (10.19)
Intrapersonal			
Pre	17.26 (6.87)	16.72 (6.01)	17.85 (4.81)
Post	19.15 (6.55)***	16.56 (6.20)	16.61 (6.20)
School Functioning			
Pre	14.29 (6.45)	12.59 (6.17)	9.85 (6.09)
Post	15.64 (6.71)**	12.69 (5.55)	9.69 (6.33)
Affective Strength			
Pre	10.98 (4.56)	9.66 (4.35)	9.04 (3.60)
Post	11.45 (4.06)	9.36 (4.67)	8.98 (5.53)
Total Score			
Pre	64.10 (22.92)	59.06 (21.22)	55.35 (15.08)
Post	69.98 (22.94)**	59.32 (21.09)	52.75 (23.87)

*$p < .05$, **$p < .01$, ***$p < .001$.

TABLE 2 Parent Ratings on the Behavioral and Emotional Ratings Scale

	Grades 1–3 ($n = 36$)	Grades 4–6 ($n = 35$)	Grades 7–8 ($n = 7$)
Interpersonal			
Pre	21.82 (6.09)	20.15 (8.22)	22.57 (5.32)
Post	24.32 (7.05)*	22.68 (8.50)*	25.43 (9.48)
Intrapersonal			
Pre	21.06 (4.90)	19.29 (5.68)	20.94 (5.17)
Post	22.74 (4.75)*	20.93 (5.19)	23.71 (5.25)
School Functioning			
Pre	15.96 (3.18)	14.16 (4.86)	16.00 (6.00)
Post	16.98 (3.60)*	14.39 (4.83)	16.49 (4.77)
Affective Strength			
Pre	13.76 (2.66)	12.48 (4.06)	13.14 (2.61)
Post	14.89 (2.36)*	13.18 (4.19)	14.10 (3.84)
Family Involvement			
Pre	19.91 (4.04)	18.77 (5.27)	20.16 (2.48)
Post	21.06 (3.90)*	20.00 (5.43)*	19.59 (4.44)
Total Score			
Pre	92.58 (16.19)	84.84 (24.07)	92.82 (18.56)
Post	99.99 (17.74)**	91.19 (24.72)	99.32 (23.39)

*$p < .05$, **$p < .01$.

$p = .035$ (see Table 2). Analysis of the Total BERS scores indicated that across all five subscales, parents of the Grades 1 through 3 students reported significant improvement. For Grades 4 through 6, parents reported significant improvements only on the dimensions of Interpersonal Strength, $t(34) = -2.25$, $p = .031$, and Family Involvement, $t(34) = -2.12$, $p = .041$; however, the levels of reported change on the Intrapersonal Strength, $t(34) = -2.08$, $p = .053$, and Total BERS scores, $t(34) = -1.99$, $p = .055$, both approximated the level of statistical significance. No improvements were found based on parent ratings of the students in Grades 7 through 8.

Student Ratings

Responses on the child self-report measure were averaged to create a total score for each child. A series of paired t tests assessing pre- and posttest scores revealed a significant change was found for the Grades 1 through 3 students, $t(63) = -3.96$, $p < .001$, although no difference over time was found for the Grades 4 through 6 or the Grades 7 through 8 students (see Table 3).

In regards to the wait-list students, no significant difference was found when their baseline self-reports were compared to those of the program participants, $t(162) = -1.69$, $p > .05$. In contrast to the program participants, paired t tests revealed that the wait-list participants did not significantly change, $t(20) = -1.67$, $p > .05$, in their pre- to posttest self-report ratings

TABLE 3 Student Self-Reports of Emotional Management Skills

	Treatment Group		
	Grades 1–3 ($n = 64$)	Grades 4–6 ($n = 57$)	Grades 7–8 ($n = 17$)
Pre	1.06 (.39)	1.33 (.39)	1.31 (.37)
Post	1.32 (.50)***	.42 (.35)	1.43 (.35)
	Comparison Group		
	Grades 1–3 ($N = 10$)	Grades 4–6 ($N = 9$)	Grades 7–8 ($N = 3$)
Pre	1.36 (.42)	1.25 (.47)	1.20 (.56)
Post	1.48 (.39)	1.41 (.36)	1.25 (.21)

***$p < .001$

(Table 3). When analyzed by grade, no change over time was found for any of the age groups on the waiting list.

DISCUSSION

Results indicated that the STEAM program, as rated by teachers, parents, and the children themselves, was effective in producing changes in emotional management skills. These positive outcomes are similar to those reported by such programs as PATHS and Second Step. However, this research demonstrated that these changes vary by age group, with the youngest children showing the most improvement. Specifically, children in Grades 1 through 3 rated themselves as improving significantly following the program, which was further supported by parent ratings that revealed improvement in all five dimensions of the BERS, and teacher ratings that revealed improvement on three of the four dimensions that were assessed by the teachers. Comparatively less improvement was shown by children in Grades 4 through 6, with a significant change on two of the five BERS dimensions, as rated by their parents. Children in Grades 7 through 8 demonstrated no improvement following the STEAM program, as measured by their self-report, and teacher and parent ratings.

These findings show evidence for the efficacy of early-intervention programs targeting children with poor emotional management skills. The potential for improvement demonstrated by the children in Grades 1 through 3 appears to be dampened even by the time children reach Grades 4 through 6. This supports Whitesell and Harter's (1996) view that interventions should occur as soon as possible before patterns of poor emotional management become ingrained. Overall, these results appear to suggest that it grows increasingly difficult to produce improvements in emotional management skills as children age.

The results of the current study also suggest difficulties in using a single instrument such as the BERS to address children's behavior across a variety of settings (i.e., home and school). Although Epstein and Sharma (1998) claimed to have designed the measure for use by parents and school professionals, our data suggest that a number of the questions assess areas of the child's functioning that may not be known to parents and teachers. In particular, only about one third of the teachers responded to all questions measuring the dimension of the child's Family Involvement. Teachers also appeared to have difficulty answering other items that were not included on the Family Involvement dimension; specifically, items 3 ("Accepts a hug"), 22 ("Enjoys a hobby"), 25 ("Accepts the closeness and intimacy of others"), and 47 ("Studies for tests"). Parents appeared to have a much better understanding of their child's functioning in all areas, and they were subsequently able to respond to all five dimensions of the BERS. The only item parents appeared to have trouble endorsing was item 29 ("Interacts positively with siblings"), which suggests that scoring allowances should be made for children who have no siblings. Further potential difficulties with the use of the BERS were illustrated by the finding that changes reported by parents were not related to the changes reported by teachers. To determine if the same children who were reported to make improvements by their teachers were also seen to make improvements by their parents, correlations on the pre- to posttest difference scores for the BERS were run. No significant correlations (range of $r = -.05$ for intrapersonal strength to $r = .22$ for school functioning) were found for the BERS total score or for any of the four subscales that were completed by parents and teachers. This perhaps reflects some of the difficulty that parents and teachers have in assessing areas of the child's life of which they are not particularly knowledgeable. More important, this finding supports the importance of multiple sources of information from the home and school, as emotion management skills may not be manifest in the same way in both environments.

The limitations of the current study include the utilization of the BERS and the high frequency of missing data that resulted from the use of this measure. That said, the omission of BERS ratings by teachers and parents for the wait-list groups cannot be seen as having enhanced the effort to assess the efficacy of the STEAM program. Although no significant baseline differences were found, it is possible that the absence of random assignment of participants to the treatment and waiting-list groups could introduce a potential bias into the sample. Another limitation of the current study that deserves mention is the small number of students in Grades 7 through 8. It would have been preferable to have a larger sample of the older age group in order to increase our confidence in the age-based effects that were demonstrated in the current study. Finally, the practice of aggregating the data across groups run by different leaders (i.e., age cohorts and total sample) could obscure material between-group variation in the STEAM program's efficacy.

Overall, the strengths of the STEAM program were the wide age range that it targeted as well as the focus on overall emotional management skills rather than just anger management. A strength of this evaluation was that it assessed change in the home and school environment and allowed for input on any behavioral changes from the children themselves. The collection of program evaluation data from multiple sources (i.e., triangulation) leads to greater confidence in the validity of the study's findings (Posavac & Carey, 2002).

Although the STEAM program and earlier curriculums such as Second Step and PATHS have been shown to be effective, there are important methodological differences that deserve further attention in the literature. Specifically, Second Step and PATHS are classroom-based programs, whereas the STEAM program was conducted with students on a pull-out basis (i.e., in a community agency). Future research should attempt to determine the relative effectiveness of both approaches. Furthermore, though the current study suggests that early-intervention emotional management programs are the most effective at producing change, future research should determine what interventions may be most appropriate for inducing change in children in Grades 4 and beyond. A longer follow-up period may also reveal the ability of such intervention programs to produce permanent changes in behavior.

ACKNOWLEDGMENT

This research was sponsored by the Waterloo Catholic Separate School Board, K-W Counseling, and the Betty Thompson Youth Centre to teach practicum students about the principles of evidence-based practice. The authors would like to thank Lisa Beck and Sarah Storry as well as the other MSW students from Wilfrid Laurier University and the BSW students from Renison College who facilitated the program and participated in the collection of data for this research. Special appreciation is extended to the parents, teachers, and principals at each of the schools that participated in the program.

REFERENCES

Achenbach, T. M., & Elderbrood, C. S. (1981). Behavior problems and competencies reported by parents of normal and disturbed children aged four through 16. *Monographs of the Society for Research in Child Development, 46*.

Akande, A. (1996). Treating anger: The misunderstood emotion in children. *Early Child Development & Care, 132,* 75–91.

Bower, E. M. (1981). *Early identification of emotionally handicapped children in schools* (3rd ed.). Springfield, IL: Charles C Thomas.

Crick, N. R. (1996). The role of overt aggression, relational aggression, and prosocial behavior in the prediction of children's future social adjustment. *Child Development, 67,* 2317–2327.

Cullinan, D., Epstein, M. H., & Kauffman, J. M. (1984). Teachers' ratings of students' behaviors: What constitutes behavior disorder in the schools? *Behavioral Disorders, 10,* 9–19.

Deffenbacher, J. L., Lynch, R. S., Oetting, E. R., & Kemper, C. C. (1996). Anger reduction in early adolescents. *Journal of Counseling Psychology, 43,* 149–157.

Dice, M. L., Jr. (1993). *Intervention strategies for children with emotional or behavioral disorders.* San Diego, CA: Singular Publishing Group, Inc.

Dunn, J., & Brown, J. (1991). Relationships, talk about feelings, and the development of affect regulation in early childhood. In J. Garber & K. A. Dodge (Eds.), *The development of emotion regulation and dysregulation.* (pp. 89–108). New York: Cambridge University Press.

Dupont, H. (1994). *Emotional development theory and applications: A neo-piagetian perspective.* Westport, CT: Praeger Publishers/Greenwood Publishing Group.

Ecton, R. B., & Feinder, E. L. (1986). *Adolescent anger control: Cognitive-behavioral techniques.* Toronto, Canada: Pergamon Press.

Eisenberg, N., Fabes, R. A., & Murphy, B. C. (1996). Parents' reactions to children's negative emotions: Relations to children's social competence and comforting behavior. *Child Development, 67,* 2227–2247.

Epstein, M. H., & Sharma, J. M. (1998). *Behavioral and emotional ratings scale: A strength based approach to assessment.* Austin, TX: Pro-Ed.

Friesen, B. J., & Osher, T. W. (1996). Involving families in change: Challenges and opportunities. In R. J. Illback & C. M. Nelson (Eds.), *Emerging school-based approaches for children with emotional and behavioral problems: Research and practice in service integration* (pp. 1–5). Binghamton, NY: Haworth Press.

Frey, K. S., Hirschstein, M. K., & Guzzo, B. A. (2000). Second step: Preventing aggression by promoting social competence. *Journal of Emotional and Behavioral Disorders, 8,* 102–112.

Garner, P. W., & Power, T. G. (1996). Preschoolers' emotional control in the disappointment paradigm and its relation to temperament, emotional knowledge, and family expressiveness. *Child Development, 67,* 1406–1419.

Greenberg, M. T., Kusche, C. A., Cook, E. T., & Quamma, J. P. (1995). Promoting emotional competence in school-aged children: The effects of the PATH curriculum. *Development and Psychopathology, 7,* 117–136.

Grossman, D. C., Neckerman, H. J., Koepsell, T. D., Liu, P. Y., Asher, K. N., Beland, K., et al. (1997). Effectiveness of a violence prevention curriculum among children in elementary school. A randomized controlled trial. *Journal of the American Medical Association, 277,* 1605–1611.

Gumora, G., & Arsenio, W. F. (2002). Emotionality, emotion regulation, and school performance in middle school children. *Journal of School Psychology, 40,* 395–413.

Illback, R. J., & Nelson, C. M. (1996). Conceptual foundations of school-based integrated services. In R. J. Illback & C. M. Nelson (Eds.). *Emerging school-based approaches for children with emotional and behavioral problems: Research and practice in service integration* (pp. 1–5). Binghamton: Haworth Press.

Moore, B., & Beland, K. (1992). *Evaluation of Second Step, pre-school-kindergarten: A violent prevention curriculum kit. Summary report*. Seattle, WA: Committee for Children.

Nelson, J. R., & Colvin, G. (1996). Designing supportive school environments. In R. J. Illback & C. M. Nelson (Eds.), *Emerging school-based approaches for children with emotional and behavioral problems: Research and practice in service integration*. (pp. 169–186). Binghamton, NY: Haworth Press.

Osher, D., & Hanley, T. V. (1996). Implications of the national agenda to improve results for children and youth with or at risk of serious emotional disturbance. In R. J. Illback & C. M. Nelson (Eds.), *Emerging school-based approaches for children with emotional and behavioral Problems: research and practice in service integration* (pp. 7–36). Binghamton, NY: Haworth Press.

Posavac, E. J., & Carey, R. G. (2002). *Program evaluation: Methods and case studies* (6th ed.). Englewood Cliffs, NJ: Prentice Hall.

Rose, S. D. (1974). *Treating children in groups: A behavioral approach*. Washington, DC: Jossey-Bass.

Schiffer, M. (1984). *Children's group therapy: Methods and case histories*. New York: Free Press.

Sukhodolsky, D. G., Solomon, R. M., & Perine, J. (2000). Cognitive-behavioral, anger-control intervention for elementary school children: A treatment outcome study. *Journal of Child & Adolescent Group Therapy, 10*, 159–170.

Whitesell, N. R., & Harter, S. (1996). The interpersonal context of emotion: Anger with close friends and classmates. *Child Development, 67*, 1345–1359.

Wilde, J. (1995). *Anger management in schools: Alternatives to student violence*. Lancaster, PA: Technomic Publishing.

Zaichkowsky, L. B., & Zaichkowsky, L. D. (1984). The effects of a school-based relaxation training program on fourth grade children. *Journal of Clinical Child Psychology, 13*, 81–85.

Zeman, J., Shipman, K., & Suveg, C. (2002). Anger and sadness regulation: Predictions to internalizing and externalizing symptoms in children. *Journal of Clinical Child & Adolescent Psychology, 31*, 393–398.

APPENDIX A

Session Topics and Objectives for both STEAM Programs

Session Topic	Temper-Taming Objectives	Taming the Dragon Objectives
Getting acquainted	• To provide structure and purpose for the group • To develop group norms, ground rules, and cohesion	• To provide structure and purpose for the group • To develop group norms, ground rules, and cohesion
2. Clues to my emotions	• To externalize temper • To determine the who, what, where and when of temper	• To identify physiological and situational "triggers" for anger and other emotions
3. Dealing with feelings	• To identify the physiological responses to emotions and temper	• To use "triggers" as a cue to reduce intensity of feelings
4. Feelings awareness	• To facilitate identification and expression of feelings	• To identify ways to deal with feelings • To increase repertoire of strategies to cope with emotions
Sometimes I wear a mask	• Concept of "being in charge" of temper through making choices • Review of sessions 1–4	• To enhance communication strategies • To illustrate that there are more ways to interpret an event or situation
Staying in control	• How not to explode • Looking critically at reactions to emotion-provoking situations • Continuation of "being in charge" of temper through making choices	• To illustrate that anger does not equal aggressive behavior • To demonstrate that choices are available in all situations
Our actions	• Staying in control • To provide opportunities to utilize coping statements to help control emotions • Making choices • Introduce and practice the concept of "self-talk"	• Staying in control • To provide opportunities to utilize coping statements to help control emotions • Making choices • Introduce and practice the concept of "self-talk"

(Continued)

Ways people handle emotions	• To understand that people handle emotions/anger in different ways • To present six different ways people handle anger • To identify their own style	• To understand that people handle emotions/anger in different ways • To present six different ways people handle anger • To identify their own style
9. Changing angry thinking	• Productive problem solving • Assist group to realize there are some situations in their lives they cannot change • To help become familiar with passive, aggressive, and assertive reactions • To present problem-solving situations	• Productive problem solving • Assist group to realize there are some situations in their lives they cannot change • To help become familiar with passive, aggressive, and assertive reactions • Discussion of positive and negative thinking
10. My responsibility	• Review concepts and attempt to integrate skills • How to get "back on track" when "old habits" kick in • To enhance the ability to take responsibility for personal actions and apologize where suitable	• Review concepts and attempt to integrate skills • How to get "back on track" when "old habits" kick in • To enhance the ability to take responsibility for personal actions and apologize where suitable
I'm in charge	• Celebrate being "in charge" of temper • Discuss the concept of complimenting others as well as receiving compliments	• Celebrate being "in charge" of temper • Discuss the concept of complimenting others as well as receiving compliments
12. Putting it all together	• To transfer skills and strategies learned in group to school setting • To develop leadership skills in children	• To transfer skills and strategies learned in group to school setting • To develop leadership skills in children

Autism Spectrum Disorders: Building Social Skills in Group, School, and Community Settings

AMIE W. DUNCAN

Cincinnati Children's Hospital Medical Center, Cincinnati, Ohio, USA

LAURA GROFER KLINGER

University of Alabama, Tuscaloosa, Alabama, USA

Adolescents diagnosed with autism spectrum disorders (ASD) face a variety of social difficulties as they interact with same-aged peers and adults in their schools and communities. Few empirically based interventions have been designed to increase social under-standing (e.g., understanding gestures and facial expressions), social interaction abilities (e.g., initiating conversation with peers), and social competence (e.g., distinguishing between teasing and joking). This article reviews the most effective strategies for increas-ing social skills in adolescents with ASD and also gives examples of how to implement these strategies in group, school, and community settings.

My big problems came in high school. That was my terrible time. Once kids start moving through puberty into adolescence, they are no longer interested in sails and kites and bike races and board games. Attention and interest turns to all things social-emotional. For me, that spelled disaster. While I understood how to be polite, and act appropriately in different situations with other kids—that is, my social functioning skills were good—I didn't feel that sense of social bonding that seems to glue kids together in their teens. (Temple Grandin, an adult with autism, discussing her high school years, cited in Grandin & Barron, 2005, p. 19)

Although individuals with autism spectrum disorders (ASD) are continually challenged by their social impairments throughout the life span, the social demands of adolescence present a particularly difficult developmental stage. For example, adolescence often requires that individuals with ASD learn more complex social rules such as understanding humor and slang, taking the perspectives of others to understand emotions and situations, and interpreting abstract language and social cues within the context of the social environment, all areas of impairment for individuals with ASD (Kasari & Rotheram-Fuller, 2007). Despite these challenges, adolescents with ASD, like their typical peers, often have a strong desire to engage in social interaction and make friends (Mesibov & Handlan, 1997; Volkmar & Klin, 1995). The purpose of this article is to discuss various group interventions for adolescents with ASD that can be used to increase social skills and facilitate social interactions with their peers in various environments. We begin with a review of the specific difficulties experienced by adolescents with ASD and then describe empirically supported interventions and the way that we have integrated them into our clinical practice.

SOCIAL IMPAIRMENTS IN ADOLESCENTS WITH AUTISM SPECTRUM DISORDER

Researchers have examined not only social skills impairments in adolescents with ASD, but also how these social difficulties may affect interactions with others and overall quality of life. Orsmond, Krauss, and Seltzer (2004) surveyed 235 adolescents and adults with ASD and found that 46% of individuals with ASD had no reciprocal friendships. They attributed the lack of friends to poor social skills that persist into adolescence. These continued social skills impairments in adolescence were documented by Church, Alisanksi, and Amanullah (2000) through a chart review of middle school and high school students seen in an autism clinic. According to clinic records, parents believed that social skills and the ability to interact with others were their adolescents' greatest challenges. Parents reported that their adolescents with ASD continued to have one-sided conversation with peers, engaged in minimal small talk with peers, displayed inappropriate and immature behavior in social situations, experienced difficulties with peer rejection due to lack of social insight, and had difficulties interpreting nonverbal and verbal communication cues.

Despite their social skills difficulties, adolescents with ASD often desire friendships and express concerns about their lack of reciprocal friendships and difficulties maintaining and sustaining friendships (Church et al., 2000). Unsurprisingly, poor social skills in ASD have been linked to significant levels of anxiety (e.g., compulsive and ritualistic behavior, irrational fears and beliefs) and depression, (e.g., increased aggression, poor relationships with parents and teachers) (Capps, Sigman, & Yirmiya, 1995; Ghaziuddin, Alessi, & Greden, 1995; Ghaziuddin, Wieder-Mikhail, & Ghaziuddin, 1998; Green, Gilchrist, Burton, & Cox, 2000; Kim, Szatmari, Bryson, Streiner, & Wilson, 2000; Leyfer et al., 2006). However, adults and adolescents with ASD who possessed well-developed abilities to interact with others were more likely to participate in various social and recreational activities (e.g., attend weekly church services, socialize with friends/neighbors weekly) (Orsmond et al., 2004). These findings suggest that adolescents with ASD desire social inter-actions, and that increased social skills are likely to provide an opportunity for more successful social interactions and improved quality of life with decreased anxiety and depression.

SOCIAL SKILLS INTERVENTIONS FOR ADOLESCENTS WITH ASD

It is critical for adolescents with ASD to be instructed on various social skills so that they can develop relationships with peers, be successful in academic and vocational settings, increase their quality of life, and combat symptoms of anxiety and depression. However, there are only a handful of empirically supported interventions for social skills and the effectiveness of these inter-ventions has been mixed (Barry et al., 2003; Bauminger, 2007a, b; Bellini, Peters, Benner, & Hopf, 2007; Charlop-Christy & Kelso, 2003; Gresham, Sugai, & Horner, 2001; Hwang & Hughes, 2000; Klinger & Williams, 2008; Krantz & McClannahan, 1993; Krasny, Williams, Provencal & Ozonoff, 2003; Lopata, Thomeer, Volker, Nida, & Lee, 2008; McConnell, 2002; Rogers, 2000; Ruble, Willis, & Crabtree, 2008; Solomon, Goodlin-Jones, & Anders, 2004; Tse, Strulovitch, Tagalakis, Meng, & Fombonne, 2007; Williams, Johnson, & Sukhodolsky, 2005). Across these studies, however, there is support for sev-eral strategies that lead to successful acquisition of social skills in individuals with ASD (see Gresham et al., 2001; Klinger & Williams, 2008; Rogers, 2000, for reviews). Klinger and Williams (2008) suggested that many successful social skills interventions utilize a "compensation" approach in which chil-dren with ASD are explicitly taught how to understand and interpret social cues and behaviors to compensate for their lack of implicit understanding of social information. Many empirically supported social skills interventions utilized similar techniques including incidental teaching, social stories and scripts, role-plays, self-monitoring, and peer-mediated activities (e.g., peer education, peer buddy). For example, Lopata and colleagues (2008) derived their social skills curriculum for high-functioning school-age children with ASD from the program *Skillstreaming* (Goldstein & McGinnis, 1997), which follows a specific stepwise procedure for teaching, modeling, role-playing, and feedback of a social skill. The specific rationale, details, and empirical support for several of these successful techniques are reviewed briefly prior to discussing their implementation in a group setting.

Incidental Teaching

Incidental teaching methods can be used within a social skills intervention to discuss social problems as they arise and also give constructive feedback about how to handle various social situations (McGee, Morrier, & Daly, 2001). For example, a therapist or teacher can point out when an adolescent with ASD has been talking about an intense interest (e.g., computer programming) for several minutes. This then gives the adult an opportunity to discuss how to initiate conversation about other topics people may be interested in (e.g., what people did over the weekend) and discuss how to recognize when others may be bored with a conversation (e.g., looking at their watch).

Social Stories and Scripts

Social stories (Gray, 1998, 2000) are short narratives that describe how to behave in social situations in a very explicit manner. Similarly, social scripts describe specific comments and questions that are appropriate in a given social situation (Barry et al., 2003; Charlop-Christy & Kelso, 2003; Krantz & McClannahan, 1993; Myles, Trautman, & Schlevan, 2004). Providing specific guidelines and rules for interacting with others not only explains a particular social situation, but also helps clarify the complex nature of the social environment and provides practical social solutions (Myles et al., 2004). For example, a social story or script may be utilized to explicitly instruct individuals with ASD on how to introduce themselves to others, how to ask for help in a classroom, how to initiate a conversation with a peer, and how to join a group of peers. Social stories and scripts are situation specific, and a variety of social stories and scripts are needed to address the individual social skills difficulties of each adolescent with ASD.

Role-Plays

Group role-plays provide an opportunity for the individual with ASD to practice a particular skill or strategy and observe others practicing the same skill (Barry et al., 2003; Goldstein & McGinnis, 1997; Klinger & Williams, 2008; Lopata et al., 2008; Ruble et al., 2008). Role-plays are typically preceded by the direct instruction of a skill (i.e., through a social story or script) so that adolescents have a foundation on which to then practice the skill. Examples of role-plays for adolescents with ASD might include how to ask a teacher a question during class, how to ask a friend to hang out over the weekend, how to initiate conversation with a peer about what they did over the weekend, and so on. For example, Barry and colleagues (2003) taught school-age children with ASD a social script for greeting other children and then had them role-play how to greet peers. Increased greeting behaviors were observed during interactions with unfamiliar peers in the clinic setting. However, parents did not report a statistically significant difference in greeting skills at home and school, suggesting that it is important to practice role-plays in various settings so that skills can generalize to different social environments (see Charlop-Christy & Kelso, 2003, for results that demonstrated generalization of conversational skills).

Self-Monitoring

Self-monitoring is an important tool that can be used to help adolescents with ASD keep track of their own progress in using appropriate social skills (see Lee, Simpson, & Shogren, 2007, for a meta-analysis on the use and effectiveness on self-management in individuals with ASD). Like role-plays, self-monitoring techniques are typically taught following direct instruction of a skill (i.e., through a social story or script). Self-monitoring can be used to track a variety of social skills including increased social interaction (e.g., the number of times an adolescent approached another person during a party) and increased appropriate social behavior (e.g., the number of times the adolescent asked a peer a question during a conversation). If an adolescent with ASD is able to monitor the proficiency with which they are utilizing certain skills in social situations, they will likely become increasingly successful at interacting with others and their self-efficacy in social situations will likely increase.

Because of increased symptoms of anxiety and depression and difficulty understanding and interpreting the emotions of others, adolescents with ASD benefit from strategies that help them to monitor their own emotions. Adolescents with ASD can learn to self-monitor their own emotions after basic education on emotion identification and coping. A picture of a thermometer can be used to demonstrate that different emotions are felt more intensely than others (e.g., annoyed is less intense than enraged) (Beebe & Risi, 2003). Reaven and colleagues (2007) used a similar technique for school-age children with ASD such that a stress-ometer was used to increase identification of anxiety symptoms and use of appropriate coping strategies (Reaven & Hepburn, 2003; Reaven et al., 2007). Adolescents can also write down the physical and mental cues associated with different emotional states on the thermometer, which can then help them determine how they are feeling (e.g., "When I am enraged my face is red and my thoughts race"). Last, coping strategies for different emotional states can be developed for each adolescent (e.g., "I need to listen to music when I'm enraged"). In addition, an emotion thermometer can be used to compare how other adolescents might feel in a particular situation and how their physical and mental cues and coping strategies may differ. Thus, emotion thermometers not only increase self-monitoring of emotions but also lead to an understanding of how others might feel in similar situations.

Peer Education

Peer education provides information (e.g., social difficulties, communication difficulties, repetitive behaviors, etc.) to students about their peers with ASD who may be in a general education classroom and/or special education classroom (Campbell, 2006; Campbell, Ferguson, Herzinger, Jackson, & Marino, 2004; Faherty, 2001; Swaim & Morgan, 2002). Results of peer education programs have been mixed. For example, Swaim and Morgan (2002) reported that children with typical development in third grade and sixth grade, who participated in a peer education program, rated a video of a child with typical development more favorably than a video of a child who displayed symptoms of ASD. However, children with typical development reported that they would likely participate in shared interests and activities with the child with ASD despite their unfavorable attitudes. In a replication of Swaim and Morgan's study, Campbell and colleagues (2004) found that children with typical development viewed the child with ASD more favorably when given both descriptive information (e.g., hobbies) and explanatory information (e.g., description of autism). In regards to issues that may affect the success or effectiveness of peer education, Campbell (2006) discussed the importance of factors such as source (e.g., likeability of individual facilitating peer education program), message (e.g., using descriptive information versus explanatory information), and the characteristics of the child with autism (e.g., appropriate vs. inappropriate social behavior).

Two of the most commonly used peer education programs are *The Sixth Sense II* (Gray, 2002) and *Understanding Friends* (Faherty, 2001). Both programs emphasize the ideas that individuals with ASD have similar abilities, interests, skills, and talents as children with typical development and encourage empathy and helping behavior. The curriculum in Understanding Friends (Faherty, 2001) consists of three main parts that include (1) discussing the idea that everyone has a different set of strengths and weaknesses; (2) participation in an experiential activity that gives exposure to the fine motor, visual, sensory, and auditory difficulties individuals with ASD face on a daily basis; and (3) an experiential activity that gives exposure to the receptive language difficulties that individuals with ASD face on a daily basis. The curriculum in The Sixth Sense II (Gray, 2002) does not provide a label of ASD but instead discusses the fact that some peers have an impairment of the sixth or social sense. It discusses common features that individuals with autism share with their peers (e.g., discussing how individuals with ASD have similar interests, strengths, and difficulties as children with typical development) and also discusses specific difficulties in social understanding and perspective-taking. Like Faherty's curriculum, this curriculum includes experiential activities that expose peers to some of the difficulties faced by students with ASD.

Peer Buddies

Peer buddies model appropriate social interaction abilities and provide feedback to adolescents with ASD regarding their own social skills (Wagner, 2001). Peer buddies can also be utilized in clinic, school (e.g., during lunch, gym class, recess), and community (e.g., during Boy Scouts) settings. In regards to choosing appropriate peer buddies, it is necessary to choose an adolescent who has well-developed social skills, has many friends, moves easily among same-age peers, has a calm personality, has a sense of humor, has empathy/helping skills, is liked by the adolescent with ASD, and is willing to be a peer buddy (Wagner, 2001). Parents or professionals should also get parental permission from the peer buddy's parents before proceeding (see Wagner, 2001, for an example of a parental permission form). Wagner (2001) recommended that a peer buddy receive peer education about ASD and suggestions about how to handle various situations that may arise (e.g., inappropriate comments, questions from other peers, etc.). The adolescent with ASD will also need an explanation regarding the purpose and function of the peer buddy (e.g., to help you make friends at Boy Scouts, to help you learn how to converse with others during drama club).

SOCIAL SKILLS GROUP INTERVENTION FOR ADOLESCENTS WITH ASD

Social skills group interventions for individuals with ASD are often conducted in a clinical setting and facilitated by psychologists, counselors, social workers, and/or therapists. Groups are also common in school settings facilitated by school counselors, special education teachers, or speech-language pathologists. There are few empirical studies examining the effectiveness of social skills groups with this population (e.g., Barry et al., 2003; Lopata et al., 2008; Ruble et al., 2008; Solomon et al., 2004) and even fewer studies that have included adolescents (e.g., Church et al., 2000; Orsmond et al., 2004; Tse et al., 2007). The authors conducted social skills groups for high-functioning adolescents (i.e., average to above-average cognitive abilities and daily living skills) with ASD in an outpatient clinic setting. Each social skills group consisted of four to six adolescents and was held bimonthly during the academic year from August through May. Therapists were graduate students earning their doctoral degrees in clinical psychology; they were supervised by a licensed psychologist. Topics that were covered in the social skills group were chosen by the adolescents with ASD or their parents and included dating, building conversation skills, making friends, managing anxiety and depression, and increasing participation in recreation and community activities. See Table 1 for a sample semester schedule. Although we don't have empirical data to support the effectiveness of our

TABLE 1 Sample Semester Schedule for Social Skills Group Intervention

- Session 1:   Get to Know Other Group Members
- Session 2:   Anxiety and Depression in Teens: How to Identify the Symptoms
- Session 3:   Anxiety and Depression in Teens: Using Relaxation, Visualization, and Deep Breathing to Cope
- Session 4:   Anxiety and Depression in Teens: Developing Individualized Coping Strategies and Putting Them Into Practice
- Session 5:   Friendships and Dating in High School: Learning the Basics
- Session 6:   Friendships and Dating in High School: Applying What You Know
- Session 7:   How to Apply and Interview for Part-Time Jobs
- Session 8:   End of Semester Party

group interventions with adolescents, we used empirically supported strategies such as incidental teaching, social stories and scripts, role-plays, and self-monitoring techniques to build social skills.

Group Structure

Because individuals with ASD often experience anxiety in new and unstructured environments, we used a daily schedule to decrease anxiety and increase flexibility (see Kunce & Mesibov, 1998). At the beginning of each social skills session, the group leaders discussed the plan for that lesson and gave each participant an individual schedule. For example, a typical schedule outline included:

1. Socialize with other group members
2. Review homework assignment
3. Teach new skill
4. Practice new skill
5. Break: Eat snack and socialize with other group members
6. Role-play new skill
7. Assign homework
8. Parent time

The above schedule was used as an outline, and more specific details and activities were added depending on the topic being discussed or the skill being taught. For example, a schedule that outlined the topic of dating might have included items such as a worksheet that discussed the advantages and disadvantages of dating and a role-play on how to ask someone on a date (see Table 2 for an example of a detailed schedule used for a session focused on dating). Homework assignments were used to review topics discussed in group or to encourage the adolescents to think about upcoming topics. For example, the homework assignment for the session on dating was to write down what would be most rewarding and most challenging about dating. The adolescents then discussed their thoughts in the group setting and were

TABLE 2 Daily Schedule for Social Skills Group on the Topic of Dating

 1. Socialize with other group members
 2. Review homework assignment (Write down what you think would be most rewarding and most challenging about dating.)
 3. Complete worksheet: "Thinking About Dating"
 4. Complete worksheet: "Advantages and Disadvantages of Dating"
 5. Break: Eat snack and socialize with other group members
 6. Complete worksheet: "How to Let Someone Know You're Interested in Them"
 7. Role-play how to show interest in members of the opposite sex
 8. Discuss how to ask someone on a date and write a social story about the topic
 9. Role-play how to ask someone on a date
10. Parent Time

free to comment or ask questions about the responses of the other group members.

When learning and also practicing new skills, written worksheets were commonly used because we found that they increased concentration and attention on the topic, increased the likelihood of remembering what was discussed, and allowed for parents to discuss the topic with the adolescent at home. Worksheets were completed as a group, with the leader reading the questions aloud and asking for comments before the adolescents wrote down their answers. Group leaders used the questions and responses from the adolescents with ASD to teach a skill or provide guidance about how to handle a particular activity.

We used popular books, movies, television shows, and articles to emphasize session content and to provide examples from which the adolescents could model behavior. For example, group members read and discussed sections from an autobiography written by Luke Jackson, an adolescent with ASD. This book, *Freaks, Geeks, and Asperger Syndrome: A User Guide to Adolescence* (Jackson, 2002), contains chapters on topics such as dating, making friends, and disclosing one's diagnosis. We used these chapters to facilitate group discussion. For example, in his chapter on dating, Luke discusses tips such as "Try to talk to the person's friends and find out what they are interested in," and "If the person you fancy is talking to you, try to listen and not interrupt them" (Jackson, 2002, p. 175). We also used video clips from several popular teen movies (e.g., *The Breakfast Club, Mean Girls*) to practice identification of other people's emotions using verbal, non-verbal, and situational cues. This was a particularly successful strategy and allowed us to evaluate the abilities of group members to not only identify emotions, but also to develop possible coping strategies that related to the particular emotion the teens in the movies displayed.

At the conclusion of each social skills session, parents were asked to join the group to discuss what topics, skills, and strategies had been discussed. The group members were encouraged to share their new skills or knowledge with their parents.

Adapting Empirically Supported Social Skills Intervention Techniques for a Group Setting

Incidental teaching. Group members were encouraged to frequently socialize with one another. The group leaders used incidental teaching methods (Wagner, 2001) to not only model appropriate conversation skills (e.g., commenting during a conversation, ending a conversation appropriately), but also to give the group members feedback about their own conversational skills in a constructive manner (e.g., how to initiate conversation about shared interests, transitioning to new topics, etc.). Group leaders also utilized incidental teaching to discuss perspective taking. For example, if an adolescent made an inappropriate comment (e.g., "Your haircut makes your ears stick out") the group leader used this as an opportunity to discuss how the comment influenced another adolescent's feelings and how to use nonverbal cues (e.g., facial expressions, body posture, eye contact, sighing) and verbal cues to understand those feelings. Group leaders also used these opportunities to discuss the subtle differences between teasing and joking around or the difference between sarcasm and humor.

Social stories and scripts. Social stories (Gray, 1998, 2000) and scripts (Barry et al., 2003; Myles et al., 2004) were used to help adolescents with ASD learn new skills by explicitly writing down how to behave in a particular social situation. For example, during the session on dating, group members wrote their own social story about how to ask someone on a date after the topic had been discussed in the group setting. We found that social stories for adolescents were often longer than typical social stories developed for younger children so that the necessary details can be adequately covered. An example of a social script or story that we wrote to explain how to ask someone on a date is described below:

> *How to Ask Someone on a Date.* When I am interested in dating a girl, I should do things to let her know that I like her. For example, I can talk to her about things she likes, compliment her, and get to know her friends better. If I decide that I want to ask the girl on a date, I should first ask my parents for permission. My parents can help me decide where I can take the girl on a date (e.g., movies) and when we can go on the date. Next, I can call the girl on the phone to ask her for a date. If she is not at home when I call, I will politely leave a message with my name and phone number so that she can call me back. If she is home when I call, I will ask her how she is doing and make small talk about things she likes to talk about for 1-2 minutes. Then, I will ask her if she would like to go to the movies with me this weekend and tell her that my parents can drive us to the movies. If she says **YES**, we will decide which movie to go to and the exact date and time of the movie. I will then let her know that I think we will have a fun time and that I will see her at school tomorrow. If she says **NO**, I will politely say that maybe we can go to the movies together another weekend and that I will see her at school tomorrow.

This social script makes the process of asking someone on a date very explicit for adolescents with ASD. For example, it discusses the steps that need to occur before asking someone on a date (i.e., talk to your parents about the specific details of going to a movie) and provides guidelines for how to respond if the girl is available to talk on the phone (i.e., ask her to go to a movie) and if the girl is not available to talk (i.e., leave a detailed phone message).

Role-plays. After creating social stories or scripts, each group member role-played the social scenario that was discussed. Our goals for using role-plays included the opportunity for group leaders to observe how proficient an adolescent has become at a skill and the opportunity for other group members to observe others implementing the skill. For example, after learning the dating script described above, each group member role-played how to ask someone on a date over the phone while a group leader played the part of the individual being asked out. Each group member was given the opportunity to practice how to leave a message when the girl he wanted to ask out was not home, how to respond when the girl did want to go on a date to the movies, and how to respond when the girl did not want to go on a date. For the session on applying for and interviewing for part-time jobs, the adolescents with ASD role-played how to ask for a job application ("I noticed that you are hiring cooks and bus boys. I am interested in these positions and was wondering if I could please have an application to fill out?"), how to clarify questions about the job application (e.g., "I have three references, but I notice you only have room for one reference. Would you prefer a previous employer?"), and how to respond to common questions that a job interviewer may ask (e.g., "My strengths are that I am a very organized person and always show up to appointments on time"). Following each role-play, constructive and positive feedback was provided by group leaders and other group members.

Self-monitoring. During sessions that focused on anxiety and depression, group members utilized an emotion thermometer to identify different intensities of an emotion, symptoms of that particular emotion, and how to cope with that emotion (see Figure 1 for an example of a completed emotion thermometer). Further, group leaders encouraged self-monitoring within sessions. For example, if an adolescent with ASD stopped participating in the discussion, put his head down on the table, and began picking his fingernails, a group leader might point out that these were the symptoms he had identified for feeling depressed on his emotion thermometer. The group leader could then discuss what coping strategies the adolescent could use to increase his mood (e.g., taking a few deep breaths, talking to a friend, etc.).

In addition to monitoring their own emotions, we found that it was important to provide adolescents with coping skills to use when they were upset. Each adolescent was encouraged to identify individualized coping

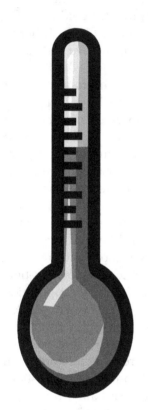

Feeling	Symptoms	Coping Strategies
Depressed *(Most Intense)*	*Crying *Thoughts Racing *Stomachache *Tired	*Write in my journal *Talk to my mom *Play a video game
Down in the Dumps *(Moderately Intense)*	*Lazy *Not Hungry *Little Stomachache *Thoughts Racing	*Walk the dog *Play a game *Call a friend
Blue *(Mildly Intense)*	*Headache *Moping Around *Don't want to talk to people *Can't sit still	*Draw or paint *Go for a walk *Help cook dinner
Sad *(Least Intense)*	*Little headache *Can still do things and talk to people *Pick my fingernails	*Take a bath *Read a book *Watch a movie

FIGURE 1 Emotion thermometer worksheet for feeling depressed.

strategies (e.g., drawing, cooking, reading, taking a bath, playing a board game, etc.) for dealing with anxiety and depression. After thinking of coping strategies, the adolescents with ASD then constructed their "emotion toolbox" (see Attwood, 2004) by collecting objects (e.g., stress ball, picture of a family member), drawing pictures, cutting out magazine pictures, or writing the coping strategies on index cards, and then placing them in a box. Each adolescent was encouraged to keep his or her "emotion toolbox" in the bedroom where it would be seen frequently and was easy to find when the adolescent was upset.

SOCIAL SKILLS INTERVENTION IN A SCHOOL SETTING

Although our social skills groups are implemented within an outpatient clinic setting, social skills groups can be implemented in a school setting with school counselors, special education teachers, or speech-language pathologists serving as group leaders. However, many middle and high schools may not have enough students with ASD to form a group. In this situation, individual instruction might be necessary. Regardless of whether skills are taught in a group or individual setting, these skills need to be practiced outside of the therapy group in "real-world" environments. This is particularly important for adolescents with ASD who have difficulty generalizing social skills learned in a clinic setting to other environments (see Barry et al., 2003). Regardless of whether the adolescent with ASD is included in the regular education classroom, receives resource services while included in the regular education classroom, or is in a special education classroom, the school setting provides opportunities for additional contact with same-age peers so that social skills can be learned, maintained, and generalized.

The success of social interactions in the school setting benefits from the inclusion of typical peers through the use of peer buddy programs, incidental teaching, and peer education (see Klinger & Williams, 2008; Wagner, 2001, for a description of each). In our clinical work, we have utilized Gray's (2002) peer education curriculum, *The Sixth Sense II*, to educate a middle-school classroom about a classmate with ASD who was in their general education classroom full-time. The student had a diagnosis of high-functioning ASD, was doing well academically, and participating in various extracurricular activities with his peers. However, the student with ASD was frequently teased for his intense interest in a particular book series and had difficulties comprehending when his peers were joking rather than teasing him. In this particular example, the student did not want to be identified as having autism or having difficulties with his social sense during the peer education, but did remain in his classroom during the presentation. Thus, *The Sixth Sense II* curriculum (Gray, 2002) seemed most appropriate as it does not label a particular child. Using this curriculum, we discussed a fictitious student named "Jack" with middle-school students:

> Jack is in 7th grade and doesn't have many friends. He seems really shy and has trouble speaking up in class and does not like to answer questions that the teacher asks. He has trouble speaking up during group projects, and while he wants to have a group of friends, he has difficulties joining in because he gets nervous he will make a mistake. However, Jack is really good in science and knows a lot about topics such as animals, space, and airplanes/jets. Lots of people make fun of Jack because he doesn't talk much, and because he seems "weird," no one ever sits with him at lunch.

Following this scenario, we asked students to describe the parts of the social sense that are hard for Jack, to identify the things that Jack is good at, and to identify ways that they could help Jack. After the peer education, the adolescent with ASD felt that his classmates understood him more and were friendlier to him than they had previously been. He also began eating lunch with two peers when he had previously eaten lunch by himself.

We conducted a similar peer education for a middle-school student with ASD who also had moderate intellectual disability and engaged in occasional motor tics when he was in the special education and general education classrooms. In this case, the adolescent's parents and teachers felt that some autism-specific peer education would be important to helping peers understand the adolescent's unusual behaviors. Thus, we adapted *The Sixth Sense II* (Gray, 2002) curriculum to educate the student's peers about autism and the student's specific autism symptoms. More specifically, classmates were informed that many people who had difficulties with the social sense also had a diagnosis of autism. The symptoms of autism were discussed in detail, and various examples were given. We then disclosed the name of one of their classmates who had autism and discussed the particular symptoms of ASD he displayed (e.g., poor eye contact, intensely interested in maps, vocal and motor tics) and specific ways to interact with him. As a result, this adolescent's classmates were more accepting of his unusual behaviors and also increased their attempts to include him in classroom activities.

SOCIAL SKILLS INTERVENTION IN A COMMUNITY SETTING

Although individuals with ASD will undoubtedly benefit from social skills interventions in the clinic and school settings, it is also critical that they receive instruction in how to engage in social interaction within the community. Research has demonstrated that participating in outside social activities leads to increased social skills and daily living skills in adolescents with ASD (see Orsmond et al., 2004).

There are many opportunities for individuals with ASD to participate in extracurricular activities through school and the community, and they should be encouraged to participate in any interesting social and recreational activities when possible. In particular it may be most beneficial to encourage participation in an activity that is related to the adolescent's intense interest or hobby, which often requires creativity and planning on the part of the parent or professional. For example, if an adolescent enjoys reading about basketball and memorizing the stats and scores of his favorite basketball players and teams, he can be encouraged to join the school's basketball team. However, because adolescents with ASD often have difficulties with fine and gross motor coordination, it may be more beneficial and enjoyable if the adolescent could assist the coach with managing the team (e.g., helping out with drills, getting necessary equipment ready, being in charge of keeping track of players' statistics, etc.). Other examples of matching adolescents' interest with a particular activity include encouraging the adolescent to join a band if they enjoy music or to join the art club if they enjoy painting and drawing. Thus, the adolescent will get the opportunity to participate in something he enjoys and will be placed in a situation where he will be interacting with adults and peers.

Although it is important to increase social interaction through participation in social and recreational activities, adolescents with ASD will likely benefit more if they are provided with the opportunity to build their social skills and learn how to interpret various social cues in different contexts. More specifically, the use of peer buddies who are also participating in the same social activity would allow the individual with ASD to benefit from the modeling of social interaction abilities and also receive feedback regarding their own social skills from the peer buddy.

In our clinical experience, we have assisted with the development of a peer buddy program for an adolescent with ASD who was involved in her church's youth group. The youth group met on Sunday mornings and Wednesday evenings but also had frequent outings such as scavenger hunts, going out to eat, going bowling, watching a movie at the group leader's house, etc. The adolescent with ASD was very reluctant to participate in any of these social activities and frequently demonstrated symptoms of anxiety and anger when her parents encouraged her participation. When the adolescent with ASD did attend these various youth group events she rarely initiated conversation, was unlikely to respond to the conversation attempts of others, and sat by herself whenever possible. Despite the fact that the adolescent had been taught these specific skills in our social skills group, she was not implementing these skills in a real world setting. The authors first decided to conduct a peer education with the youth group that the adolescent with ASD did not attend. More specifically, the authors utilized *The Sixth Sense II* (Gray, 2002) but also disclosed the adolescent's diagnosis and discussed the specific symptoms that the adolescent often displayed. The participants in the youth group had many questions, and these were addressed in great detail with the focus on how to facilitate social interaction with the adolescent with ASD (e.g., call her on the phone to invite her to social activities, etc.).

After the peer education had been completed, the mother of the adolescent with ASD expressed interest in also choosing a member of the youth group as a peer buddy. One particular girl stood out as a good candidate for a peer buddy because she was very friendly, socialized with several adolescents in the youth group, had expressed empathy and concern for the adolescent with ASD during the peer education, and had well-developed social skills. In addition, the adolescent with ASD also liked the potential peer buddy because they shared an interest in the same television show. When permission was obtained from the peer buddy and the peer buddy's parents, the authors trained the mother of the adolescent with ASD on how to provide guidance, education, and support for the peer buddy. More specifically, the authors discussed that the mother should review common social difficulties her adolescent with ASD encountered and give specific examples of how to appropriately model or give feedback about these social difficulties. For example, the adolescent with ASD rarely made eye contact when conversing with others, and the peer buddy could help increase this skill by gently reminding the adolescent with ASD to look at her when talking or give her feedback about her eye contact after she had conversed with others. The mother was encouraged to check in with the peer buddy to ensure that she was effectively modeling appropriate social skills and felt comfortable working with the adolescent with ASD. The authors also encouraged the mother to provide the peer buddy with occasional reinforcement for her effort (e.g., book, gift certificate to the movies).

Thus far, the adolescent has benefitted immensely from the peer education at her youth group and the peer buddy. The adolescent with ASD frequently attends various youth group activities and also occasionally talks to her peer buddy on the phone. Her parents also reported that she seems to be experiencing less anxiety and anger regarding attending youth group.

SUMMARY AND CONCLUSIONS

Adolescents with ASD are faced with increasingly complex social situations that require them to decipher a variety of social cues despite their social impairments. In addition, though adolescents with ASD often experience anxiety, depression, and low self-esteem as a result of their social deficits, those adolescents with ASD who have increased social skills are more likely to have reciprocal friendships and participate in social and recreational activities (Orsmond et al., 2004). Thus, it is necessary for social skill interventions to be implemented in the clinic, school, and community settings to increase learning, maintenance, and generalization of social skills so that adolescents can successfully transition to other developmental stages including secondary education and employment. Despite the clinical need for providing social skills interventions for adolescents with ASD, there is a dearth of empirical literature supporting the effectiveness of these interventions. Future research is clearly needed to develop and assess the efficacy of social skills interventions for adolescents with ASD.

REFERENCES

Attwood, T. (2004). *Exploring feelings: Cognitive behaviour therapy to manage anxiety*. Arlington, TX: Future Horizons.

Barry, T. D., Klinger, L. G., Lee, J. M., Palardy, N., Gilmore, T., & Bodin, S. D. (2003). Examining the effectiveness of an outpatient clinic-based social skills group for high functioning children with autism. *Journal of Autism and Developmental Disorders, 33*, 685–701.

Bauminger, N. (2007a). Brief report: Group social-multimodal intervention for HFASD. *Journal of Autism and Developmental Disorders, 37*, 1605–1615.

Bauminger, N. (2007b). Brief report: Individual social-multi-modal intervention for HFASD. *Journal of Autism and Developmental Disorders, 37*, 1593–1604.

Beebe, D. W., & Risi, S. (2003). Treatment of adolescents and young adults and high-functioning autism or Asperger syndrome. In M. A. Reinecke, F. M. Dattilio, & A. Freeman (Eds.), *Cognitive therapy with children and adolescents: A casebook for clinical practice* (2nd ed., pp. 369–401). New York: Guilford Press.

Bellini, S., Peters, J., Benner, L., & Hopf, A. (2007). A meta-analysis of school-based social skill interventions for children with autism spectrum disorders. *Remedial and Special Education, 28*, 153–162.

Campbell, J. M. (2006). Changing children's attitudes toward autism: A process of persuasive communication. *Journal of Developmental and Physical Disabilities, 18*, 251–272.

Campbell, J. M., Ferguson, J. E., Herzinger, C. V., Jackson, J. N., & Marino, C. A. (2004). *Research in Developmental Disabilities, 25*, 321–339.

Capps, L., Sigman, M., & Yirmiya, N. (1995). Self-competence and emotional understanding in high-functioning children with autism. *Development and Psychopathology, 1*, 137–149.

Charlop-Christy, M. H., & Kelso, S. E. (2003). Teaching children with autism conversational speech using a cue card/written script program. *Education and Treatment of Children, 26*, 108–127.

Church, C., Alisanski, S., & Amanullah, S. (2000). The social, behavioral, and academic experiences of children with Asperger's syndrome. *Focus on Autism and Other Developmental Disabilities, 15*, 12–20.

Faherty, C. (2001). *Understanding friends: A program to educate children about differences, and to foster empathy.* Retrieved July 13, 2008, from University of North Carolina, TEACCH Website: http://www.teacch.com/understandingfriends.html

Ghaziuddin, M., Alessi, N., & Greden, J. F. (1995). Life events and depression in children with pervasive developmental disorders. *Journal of Autism and Developmental Disorders, 25*, 495–502.

Ghaziuddin, M., Wieder-Mikhail, W., & Ghaziuddin, N. (1998). Comorbidity of Asperger syndrome: A preliminary report. *Journal of Intellectual Disability Research, 42*, 179–283.

Goldstein, A. P., & McGinnis, E. (1997). *Skillstreaming the adolescent: New strategies and perspectives for teaching prosocial skills.* Champaign, IL: Research Press.

Grandin, T., & Barron, S. (2005). *The unwritten rules of social relationships.* Arlington, TX: Future Horizons.

Gray, C. (1998). Social stories and comic strip conversations with students with Asperger syndrome and high-functioning autism. In E. Schopler, G. B. Mesibov, & L. J. Kunce (Eds.), *Asperger syndrome or high functioning autism?* (pp. 167–198).New York: Plenum Press.

Gray, C. (2000). *The new social story book.* Arlington, TX: Future Horizons.

Gray, C. (2002). *The sixth sense II.* Arlington, TX: Future Horizons.

Green, J., Gilchrist, A., Burton, D., & Cox, A. (2000). Social and psychiatric functioning in adolescents with Asperger syndrome compared with conduct disorder. *Journal of Autism and Developmental Disorders, 30,* 279–293.

Gresham, F. M., Sugai, G., & Horner, R. H. (2001). Interpreting outcomes of social skills training for students with high-incidence disabilities. *Council for Exceptional Children, 67,* 331–344.

Hwang, B., & Hughes, C. (2000). The effects of social interactive training on early social communicative skills of children with autism. *Journal of Autism and Developmental Disorders, 30,* 331–343.

Jackson, L. (2002). *Freaks, geeks, and Asperger syndrome: A user guide to adolescence.* London: Jessica Kingsley Publishers.

Kasari, C., & Rotheram-Fuller, E. (2007). Peer relationships of children with autism: Challenges and interventions. In E. Hollander & E. Anagnostou (Eds.), *Clinical manual for the treatment of autism* (pp. 235–258).Washington, DC: American Psychological Association.

Kim, J. A., Szatmari, P., Bryson, S. E., Streiner, D. L., & Wilson, F. (2000). The prevalence of anxiety and mood problems among children with autism and Asperger disorder. *Autism, 4,* 117–132.

Klinger, L. G., & Williams, A. (2008). Cognitive behavioral interventions in students with autism spectrum disorders. In M. J. Mayer, R. VanAcker, J. E. Lochman, & F. M. Gresham (Eds.), *Cognitive behavioral interventions for students with emotional/behavioral disorders* (pp. 296–328).New York: Guilford.

Krantz, P. J., & McClannahan, L. E. (1993). Teaching children with autism to initiate to peers: Effects of a script-fading procedure. *Journal of Applied Behavior Analysis, 26,* 121–132.

Krasny, L., Williams, B. J., Provencal, S., & Ozonoff, S. (2003). Social skills interventions for the autism spectrum: Essential ingredients and a model curriculum. *Child and Adolescent Psychiatry, 12,* 107–122.

Kunce, L. J. & Mesibov, G. B. (1998). Educational approaches to high-functioning autism and Asperger Syndrome. In E. Schopler, G. B. Mesibov, & L. J. Kunce (Eds.), *Asperger syndrome or high functioning autism?* (pp. 227–261). New York: Plenum Press.

Lee, S. H., Simpson, R. L., & Shogren, K. A. (2007). Effects and implications for self-management for students with autism: A meta-analysis. *Focus on Autism and Other Developmental Disabilities, 22,* 2–13.

Leyfer, O. T., Folstein, S. E., Bacalman, S., Davis, N. O., Dinh, E., Morgan, J., et al. (2006). Comorbid psychiatric disorders in children with autism: Interview development and rates of disorders. *Journal of Autism and Developmental Disorders, 36,* 849–861.

Lopata, C., Thomeer, M. L., Volker, M. A., Nida, R. E., & Lee, G. K. (2008). Effectiveness of a manualized summer social treatment program for high-functioning children with autism spectrum disorders. *Journal of Autism and Developmental Disorders, 38,* 890–904.

McConnell, S. R. (2002). Interventions to facilitate social interaction for young children with autism: Review of available research and recommendations for educational intervention and future research. *Journal of Autism and Developmental Disorders, 32,* 351–372.

McGee, G. G., Morier, M. J., & Daly, T. (2001). The Walden early childhood programs. In J. S. Handleman & S. L. Harris (Eds.), *Preschool education programs for children with autism* (2nd ed., pp. 157–190). Austin, TX: Pro-Ed.

Mesibov, G. B., & Handlan, S. (1997). Adolescents and adults with autism. In D. J. Cohen & F. R. Volkmar (Eds.), *Handbook of autism and pervasive developmental disorders* (2nd ed., pp. 309–322). New York: John Wiley & Sons.

Myles, B. S., Trautman, M. L., & Schelvan, R. L. (2004). *The hidden curriculum: Practical solutions for understanding unstated rules in social situations.* Shawnee Mission, KS: Autism Asperger Publishing Co.

Orsmond, G. I., Krauss, M. W., & Seltzer, M. M. (2004). Peer relationships and social and recreational activities among adolescents and adults with autism. *Journal of Autism and Developmental Disorders, 34,* 245–256.

Reaven, J., Blakely-Smith, A., Nichols, S., Dasari, M., Flanigan, E., & Hepburn, S. (2007). *Cognitive-behavioral group treatment for anxiety symptoms in children with high-functioning autism spectrum disorders.* Paper presented at the International Meeting for Autism Research, Seattle, WA, May 2007.

Reaven, J., & Hepburn, S. (2003). Cognitive-behavioral treatment of obsessive-compulsive disorder in a child with Asperger syndrome: A case report. *Autism, 7,* 145–164.

Rogers, S. J. (2000). Interventions that facilitate socialization in children with autism. *Journal of Autism and Developmental Disorders, 35,* 399–409.

Ruble, L., Willis, H., & Crabtree, V. M. (2008). Social skills group therapy for autism spectrum disorders. *Clinical Case Studies, 7,* 287–300.

Solomon, M., Goodlin-Jones, B. L., & Anders, T. F. (2004). A social adjustment enhancement intervention for high functioning autism, Asperger's syndrome, and pervasive developmental disorder NIS. *Journal of Autism and Developmental Disorders, 34,* 649–668.

Swaim, K. F., & Morgan, S. B. (2002). Children's attitudes and behavioral intentions toward a peer with autistic behaviors: Does a brief educational intervention have an effect? *Journal of Autism and Developmental Disorders, 32,* 195–205.

Tse, J., Strulovitch, J., Tagalakis, V., Meng, L., & Fombonne, E. (2007). Social skills training for adolescents with Asperger syndrome and high-functioning autism. *Journal of Autism and Developmental Disorders, 37,* 1960–1968.

Volkmar, F. R., & Klin, A. (1995). Social development in autism: Historical and clinical perspectives. In S. Baron-Cohen, H. Tager-Flusberg, & D. J. Cohen (Eds.), *Understanding other minds: Perspectives from autism* (pp. 40–55). New York: Oxford University Press.

Wagner, S. (2001). *Inclusive programming for middle school students with autism.* Arlington, TX: Future Horizons.

Williams, S. K., Johnson, C., Sukhodolsky, D. G. (2005). The role of the school psychologist in the inclusive education of school-age children with autism spectrum disorders. *Journal of School Psychology, 43,* 117–136.

Part II: Issues Around Instruction and Dissemination of Evidence-Based Group Work in Practice Settings

The Andragogy of Evidence-Based Group Work: An Integrated Educational Model

DAVID E. POLLIO

University of Alabama School of Social Work Tuscaloosa, Alabama, USA

MARK J. MACGOWAN

Florida International University, Miami, Florida, USA

Despite advances in group work education and in teaching about evidence-based practice (EBP), there has been little discussion about how to integrate EBP into existing educational models and how education about EBP can add to the effectiveness of group work practice. This article advances instruction in group work through articulating EBP within integrated instructional models. Each model consists of five elements—theory, evidence, group models, practice situation, and supervision—woven together in two ways. In one, EBP is conceptualized within an integrated instructional model that suggests that all elements are essential in education to advancing effective group work. In the second, a developmental instructional model articulates how these elements are delivered in teaching, which may be differentially applied based on the level of knowledge, skill, and experience of the learner. Through these models, the authors demonstrate how evidence-based group work principles integrate with skill development in the classroom, and how both can help to improve practice behaviors in group.

Educating social workers in group work is a challenging task, in part because organizing teaching in a classroom requires a difficult balancing act between imparting knowledge and skill building in a manner that promotes sophisticated use of both in developing and leading groups. Traditionally, group work texts have focused primarily on didactic content, often organized around stages of group development interspersed with case examples. The balance between knowledge building and skill building in the classroom is frequently addressed through combining a focus on content with a series of experiential, problem-based learning exercises.

The task of balancing content with skill building in teaching group work is further complicated by the recent move toward evidence-based practice (EBP). With its focus on developing critical thinking skills, and its use of increasingly sophisticated tools for accessing information, the EBP movement has fundamentally changed our ability to incorporate a variety of evidence into the classroom and the clinical process. This adds a third and fourth element to the balance in the classroom: teaching the critical thinking skills (including the use of new technologies) and the ability to interpret and apply research related to specific issues identified by the student practitioner. This balancing act is further influenced by the specifics of the classroom, changing radically from the typical semester-long master's level class to one-day workshops for experienced clinicians.

The challenge of incorporating EBP has not been lost on group work educators. Increasingly, material on the EBP process has been available through new texts, community trainings, and presentations at conferences. This material generally focuses on the EBP process itself by introducing learners to the ideas and techniques of the approach. However, these sources have been developed without a consistent focus on how EBP is integrated within traditional educational models, and how training in EBP might serve to add to the effectiveness of group work practice.

The purpose of this article is to improve instruction in group work through conceptualizing EBP within an integrated instructional model. Teaching students and community practitioners critical thinking skills that lead to incorporating best available evidence into practice has the potential for improving group work, while increasing our ability to generate new evidence, thus improving our instruction, in an iterative process.

In developing this instructional model, the focus is not on presenting the incorporation of evidence as a panacea, or a "new paradigm" (as has been argued previously, cf. Howard, McMillan, & Pollio, 2003), but rather on how integration of best available evidence can support decision making about theories, group models, and specific practice situations. Further, building on Straus and colleagues' work in evidence-based medicine (Straus, Richardson, Glasziou, & Haynes, 2005), evidence as conceptualized here is relevant to background knowledge (e.g., including information gained in the classroom) and foreground knowledge (e.g., information gained around identifying a specific issue in practice). Instruction around how knowledge, critical thinking, and clinical skills might combine is conceptualized around a dynamic model, where the interrelationship among these factors can lead to improved decision making at group model and micro-practice levels.

In developing these concepts, we revisit the context of EBP, defining what constitutes evidence, as well as the critical thinking skills necessary to identifying evidence relevant to the specific question. Building on these definitions, we present our instructional model. Key to this model is the interrelationships among theory, evidence, group models, practice, and supervision and the dynamic nature of these constructs as they proceed over time. Having defined this model, we consider how it relates to the teaching of group work, including a focus on the andragogy of instruction. Following this, we present specific teaching skills, as well as a discussion of how these concepts might be organized in a curriculum or workshop.

CONCEPTUALIZING EBP

In beginning this task, it is necessary to begin where so many other discussions start, with defining the elements of EBP as they are used here. Defining what constitutes evidence, and how different types of information are valued has a clear impact on how evidence is integrated into practice decisions. For example, if evidence is conceptualized narrowly as that developed in rigorous research (e.g., through randomized clinical trials), the focus of evidence-based education can be organized clearly around content, and the learning task would be more heavily didactic in nature.

However, it is our position that this approach to defining evidence is, though simpler to develop inclusion and exclusion criteria, far less useful to clinicians, and thus minimizes the impact of EBP on practice. We have each argued separately (Pollio, 2006; Macgowan, 2008; and are not alone in this) that evidence is better understood as any consistent collection of knowledge, and that incorporating evidence into practice focuses around identifying the best available evidence through locating and evaluating relevant information based on a consistent metric around validity, impact, and applicability of the literature. This implies a consumer of research who is sophisticated in asking good questions (critical thinking) and interpreting evidence.

Key to this more open approach to inclusion of evidence is the knowledge that, regardless of our preferences for creating standardized models, each clinical intervention is, to some extent, unique. Further, in very few instances are models available that provide a close fit with the situation. Rather, as we have each argued previously, the task of the clinician is to act as a consumer of the evidence, being able to take what is known and translate it to the group itself and to the individual situation.

The rationale for this approach is painfully obvious. Regardless of the evidence, the clinician, the client, or any context; in the clinical moment something has to be said or done. Whether it is informed by "practice wisdom" or "evidence" or "theory" or even a "guess," something happens—effective or not, applicable or less so. For the educator, this represents a key challenge, namely, how do we create the knowledge and skills to provide the clinician with materials to make a maximally effective response? In essence, we are talking about integrating the elements of theory, group models, and evidence to increase the probability that how the clinician responds will be appropriate and useful. Further, the focus on evaluating one's own practice in EBP lends a developmental aspect to this process—systematic accumulation of our own decisions has the added benefit of improving our likelihood of making an effective response over time.

The underlying rationale for integrating a variety of approaches is further complicated in group work education. Unlike in dyads, leading a group requires interpreting the context of multiple clients, further complicating the algebra of which response is most appropriate (or even, whether a response is necessary at all). Fortunately for the practitioner (if less so for the educator), there is a large and sophisticated literature on group processes to aid in making decisions in groups. Thus, our definition of evidence includes not just clinical interventions, but also a knowledge of the impact of dynamics such as group process and structures, group leadership, member roles, and other factors.

To summarize, evidence, as used here, is any systematic collection of information. Further, building on our previous points, evidence is evaluated as it "yields documentary support for the conclusion that a practice or service has a reasonable probability of effectiveness" (Cournoyer, 2004, p. 14). For this discussion, information is located and evaluated to identify the "best available evidence," with research of greater rigor interpreted concurrently with its impact and match to the situation, then implemented in a consistent manner and evaluated to provide more information for later efforts.

From an educational perspective, key to this is the ability to develop critical thinking skills. In the EBP process, this includes four stages: (1) formulate an answerable practice question, (2) search for evidence, (3) critically review the evidence, and (4) and apply the evidence and evaluate (Macgowan, 2008). In integrating and applying best available evidence to the specific clinical process, the practitioner acts as a scientist, formulating and testing hypotheses in the clinical situation.

This idea of the clinician as a scientist, testing out solutions derived from best available evidence and using the results from testing a hypothesis to guide further inquiry, has an important impact on the way we conceptualize the interventive process (and hence the educational one). Similarly, practice has also been described not as a linear process, but rather an iterative one. This point has been made repeatedly in the group work literature (e.g., Yalom & Leszcz, 2005). In integrating the parallel ideas of science and practice as developmental processes, we can begin to construct a model that is dynamic in nature and that integrates the "scientist" and "practitioner" together in a complementary manner into an integrated instructional model. This is the task of the next section.

INTEGRATING THEORY, EVIDENCE, AND MODELS INTO PRACTICE SITUATIONS

In conceptualizing our integrated instructional model, we return to the balancing act described in the introduction to help identify the elements of this dynamic model. The first piece of the model is based on the didactic material traditionally included in group work instruction. Conceptually, this consists of two elements, (1) theory and (2) group models. The third element is, not surprisingly, (3) evidence. The fourth and final element builds from the idea that the educational process leads to the development of clinical skill, which are played out in (4) the practice situation. We first define and discuss these elements, then present how these elements interact in a dynamic process.

In defining these elements, it is important to note that the examples provided are neither exhaustive nor do they indicate a set of recommendations. As we emphasize in the section on teaching from the integrated model, decisions on the specific focus for each element is a perquisite of the instructor. Further, inclusion of material is going to vary based on the length of the instruction, the type of students and their educational level, and the specific outcomes for instruction.

Theory

A theory may be defined as "a set of interrelated constructs (concepts), definitions, and propositions that present a systematic view of phenomena by specifying relations among variables, with the purpose of explaining and predicting the phenomena" (Kerlinger, 1986, p. 9). For group work, theories can be understood at two levels. Overarching theories are constructed to describe and predict human behavior based on a series of propositions. For group work education, theories of this type that are often taught are behavioral, psychodynamic, and systems. These type theories represent organizing principles for interpreting a broad variety of situations and relationships.

A second set of theories relate to phenomena in groups or human interactions, which are often collected under the label of "group dynamics." These can include theories related to the groups themselves (such as group development or group processes) or specific actions within groups by individuals (such as group leadership). This level also can include theories related to intergroup relations, such as social comparison or relative deprivation theories, or the way in which individuals identify with groups in the social environment, such as social identity theory (cf. Cartwright & Zander, 1968; or Forsyth, 2009, for reviews of group dynamics theories).

Although it is not the intent of this discussion to include or exclude specific theories from an educational perspective, there are a number of other theories that would be appropriate conceptualized as either overarching or specific theories. Examples of these would include feminism, theories related to race and culture, and others from the social psychological and sociological literature.

Group Model

In discussing group models, we include approaches to group work, manualized or otherwise-defined groups, and techniques. Approaches to group work often emerge from a value-driven perspective, or are developed based on theories focused on describing specific phenomena. An example of a value-driven approach is strength-based group work. An example of a theory-driven approach would be mutual aid, which draws from interactional theory.

Manualized or systematically described groups often draw from, or are developed from, research. An example of this type group would be cognitive-behavioral therapy (Petrocelli, 2002; Rose, 2004). Cognitive-behavioral groups are also drawn from behavioral theory. Another popular manualized intervention is psychoeducation. Psychoeducation groups have been developed for a variety of specific populations and problems and combine elements of mutual aid, educational, and problem-solving approaches (Pollio, Brower, & Galinsky, 2000).

Techniques may be considered discrete and circumscribed and are goal oriented, planned actions undertaken by the group worker (Sheafor & Horejsi, 2006). Examples include specific actions manipulating group conditions to maximize group member engagement or cohesion, or the use of rounds to increase members' participation. Techniques may derive from a particular intervention or group approach, such as those described above, or they may be atheoretical. However, they may be used by the group work in the moment to manage a particular group concern or to maximize group conditions to enhance group process.

Evidence

We have already defined evidence as any systematic collection of information. Returning to the concept that all interventions are probabilistic, evidence is incorporated into the intervention process to increase the likelihood of effectiveness relative to unsystematic clinical intuition. Thus, evidence of any rigor constitutes a likely improvement on instinct.

One aspect of evidence from an educational perspective is to teach the evidence on which our traditional knowledge base is built. This "background knowledge" (Straus et al., 2005) is the cadre of information offered to students through classroom teaching and assigned readings on group work.

Although a foundation, the background knowledge is limited because it does not readily answer the vexing practice questions and situations students meet in the field. This second knowledge, foreground, is the knowledge derived from formulating and answering questions about specific practice circumstances encountered. Students encounter opportunities to develop this latter knowledge in their field placements. New group workers typically have only background knowledge, but as experience develops, more is drawn from foreground knowledge (Straus et al., 2005). Knowledge can come from many sources including texts, quantitative and qualitative research studies, expert opinion, and the results of personal practice evaluations (Cournoyer, 2004; Pollio, 2002, 2006).

However, knowledge itself is not evidence, but becomes so when there is a reasonable probability that the information applied will be effective (Cournoyer, 2004). It becomes the best evidence, or best available evidence, when the evidence is systematically acquired and critically reviewed for its research merit, clinical impact, and applicability to the group situation (as part of a four-stage process, see Macgowan, 2008). As accountable professionals, social workers must engage in such a critical process to evaluate all information/evidence—even material labeled "best practice" or "evidence based." Although such material may be rigorous and impactful, it may not be applicable to the group situation. For example, the "best practice" may require special training that the group worker lacks. Thus, we need to continue to teach from the traditional knowledge base and help students to learn from their practice circumstances, but do so critically. It is incumbent on educators and practitioners to be accountable to the quality of knowledge and evidence, to know the difference and strive for the best available evidence.

Practice Situation

The practice situation represents the opportunity to implement the integrated model to specific situations. This can be within classroom situations (such as group simulations) but more frequently refers to actual behaviors within groups within the agency (including practicum and postgraduate practice). Building on the other elements of the model, clinical skills are developed in the context of the practice situation. In the practice situation, theory, group models, and evidence are judiciously and skillfully applied and their effects evaluated. Workers need to make decisions about what theory, model, or evidence applies, and if and how these should be adapted to the particular group situation. In addition, the effects of applying these elements in practice require the use of evaluative skills, to assess whether desired results were achieved. The practice situation may be fertile ground for developing clinical skill as long as there are essential ingredients for success, namely, sufficient didactic material to draw upon, nimble critical thinking, and sound supervision or consultation.

Integrated Instructional Model

To this point, we have discussed the elements as if each were easily separable from the other. This is clearly not the case; the links among the various elements have unique or reciprocal influence on their potential utility in practice situations, as well as in making choices on what gets included in group work instruction. Thus, it is more useful to integrate the elements into a single construct, which will have utility to clinical decision making and to instruction.

Figure 1 presents this model. In examining the model, we are conceptualizing it at two levels. First, the model represents a dynamic construct of the intervention process itself. The interrelationships among the elements provide information relevant to choosing group models and in making choices within the practice situation. Further, the model helps guide the instructional process. As we discuss in the subsequent section, the elements provide organizing areas for didactic learning, whereas the specified relationships provide direction for discussing the process. In this section, we discuss the model as illustrating the intervention process, whereas in the subsequent section the model will be used to organize instruction.

The focus of the dynamic model is on the specific practice situation. In choosing to present the intervention process from a dynamic process, we are making the decision to move away from a more linear construct. Thus, instead of taking each situation as something with an identifiable beginning, middle, and end stage, we are seeking to understand practice as a series of events that are tied together through a series of loops—that each practice

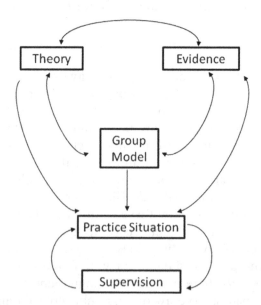

FIGURE 1 Dynamic Construction of Intervention and Instructional Process.

situation incorporates the elements, and that the history and interrelationships proceed and change (and hopefully improve) over time, with and across groups.

In one sense, the elements of theory, group model, and evidence exist within the practitioner, serving to support and guide the choices made by the group worker in each situation. The elements of theory and group model are essentially static in the practice situation. The practitioner enters each situation with the background framework of his or her theoretical approach to practice, and the model that drives the group.

Given the more fluid definition advocated in this article, evidence takes a more dynamic role in the practice situation. On one level, the group worker has the knowledge of evidence for the choices he or she makes that is brought to the situation. In this sense, evidence functions in a similar manner to theory and group model. However, given a critical thinking lens, the group worker makes his or her response based on critical thinking, namely a hypothesis on the results of the intervention. The response by the group or group member provides evidence as to whether the intervention has had the anticipated impact. This "single-system" approach can then be used as evidence to inform future practice situations—thus, the element of evidence represents an ongoing process.

The final loop in Figure 1, supervision, represents the opportunity to receive feedback from a supervisor or colleague, presumably one with either greater experience or an outside view or both. Similar to theory and group model, supervision does not have the ability to be given within the practice situation (a rare exception would be live supervision). However, separate from all the other elements, supervision involves a dynamic process taking place across multiple practice situations. Conceptually, it includes a discussion of the situation in light of the hypothesis and intervention within the practice situation and an opportunity to reflect on the other conceptual elements.

EBP AND ANDRAGOGY: TEACHING GROUP WORK

Key to teaching group work is the assumption that the learner is an adult, and is capable of participating in the educational process, rather than a more passive learning approach—thus our use of the term *andragogy*, as opposed to *pedagogy* (Merriam, 2001). Although this has been discussed in greater depth in previous work on teaching macro practice (Bricout, Pollio, Edmond, & Moore-McBride, 2008), the focus of andragogy, as we use the term here, is on the concept of the reflective practitioner, first espoused by Schön (1983, 1987) and later Schipper (1999). The reflective practitioner, rather than merely implementing theories or models, develops hypotheses (labeled "reflection in action"; Borduas,Gagnon, Lacoursiere, & Laprise, 2001), which then culminates in "knowledge in action."

Thus, the purpose of instruction in group work is to engage in a mutual process with the student focusing on creating the knowledge, skills, and values leading to becoming a reflective practitioner—an individual who uses knowledge and skills to engage in a dynamic process to continually improve the ability to function in a practice situation. Rather than conceptualizing instruction as being focused on imparting knowledge, or the ability to articulate specific models or theories, we proceed from our feedback model and the concept of reflective practitioner in andragogy to envision classroom instruction as aimed at facilitating the creation within each student of an articulated practice philosophy unique to that individual. Further, we believe that the philosophy created in the classroom represents the beginning of a dynamic growth process; that is, continuously testing the philosophy within the practice situation, incorporating new knowledge, and increasing the sophistication of critical thinking through hypothesis testing in the group situation and through supervision.

So, how is this relatively complex product of group work taught? Although some of the teaching about the content of evidence and the process of acquiring, evaluating, and applying it involves a didactic approach, the teaching is best facilitated through a problem-based learning/practice-based learning (PBL) approach. More fully described below, PBL may be defined as "an instructional method that encourages learners to apply critical thinking, problem-solving skills, and content knowledge to real-world problems and issues" (Levin, 2001, p. 1). PBL is based on a consistent understanding that didactic knowledge is necessary to advanced skills, but not sufficient unless paired with application in simulations in the classroom and practice in real-world settings.

In examining this teaching approach, this instructional model conceptualizes the classroom in much the same way as group work conceptualizes the practice situation—namely the traditional phases of beginning, middle, and end. Figure 2 presents the elements of the instructional model.

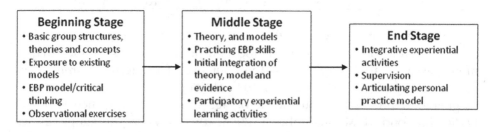

FIGURE 2 Stages of Classroom Instruction.

EBP = evidence-based practice.

This stage-based model can be understood on two levels. First, it is an ordering of the competencies leading to basic skills in group work. On this level, the competencies are cumulative—each set includes basic knowledge required to take best advantage of those in the next stage—but do not require to be taught within the same context. Thus, the model can be incorporated across an educational process, including introduction of beginning-phase skills in introductory classes, middle-phase skills in a group work class, and possibly end-phase competencies such as an initial integrated practice statement as part of a final semester practice class. It can also be used to identify competencies for individual skill-building workshops. For example, if the instructor is designing a master class for postgraduate practitioners and the audience can be anticipated to have extensive group work exposure, the instruction might focus on end-stage competencies, such as taking advantage of supervision.

At the more basic level, the stage-based model takes a task-group-focused lens to the educational process. The instructor takes the classroom situation and decides how to develop the competencies to the group. In this sense, the model provides the developmental context through which PBL is used to acquire competencies. As the tasks increase in complexity, the approach to acquiring skills increases in terms of student participation, and in terms of the complexity of the tasks and problems set before them. Again, we return to the group development literature, in that the purpose of the role of instructor (group leader) is to give away the power of the group as much as possible, making the students responsible for their individual learning. From the previous section, this is an adult-learner approach to andragogy.

In returning to the model, in the beginning phase, students learn basic definition of groups and theories, are presented with common evidence-based models, and begin learning the EBP model and evaluation skills. This phase exposes students to the first three elements described in the previous section. As the focus of the beginning phase is on introduction and setting the context, the primary educational activities are didactic and observational—students do not yet have the context to apply skills. However, learning by observing other practitioners do their work has the potential for beginning to integrate how these skilled practitioners integrate their own skills. This is not to argue that observational activities should be passive in nature. Rather, students should observe and then discuss the observations and identify generally the skills successfully displayed (and where they are unsuccessful, which may be of greater importance), and specifically how the observed skills may support their efforts to acquire their own set.

In the middle phase, students continue to develop their knowledge around the theories and models. Exposure to these elements is integrated with an emerging ability to evaluate critically the evidence supporting a particular theory or model. It is also worth noting that this phase includes the beginning of developing an understanding and incorporation of group process as part of the group model construct. Using the evidence-based group work model (Macgowan, 2008) allows an increasing ability to incorporate these skills and helps create greater depth in the understanding of specific groups and models. In looking back on the model in Figure 1, it is during this middle phase that we begin to see the dynamic interplay among the first three elements of the model.

In terms of classroom activities, at this middle phase the emphasis moves from didactic and observational toward participatory. The student is assumed to be able to acquire and evaluate knowledge without the direct input from the instructor. Thus, lectures become fewer, essentially limited to some of the more complex elements that may require some specific explanation of methods beyond that which can reasonably be expected from the students, and the classroom becomes more participatory. This can take several forms. Students might be expected to present information around assigned elements integrating their critical thinking skills and individual perspectives to explore the concepts in greater depth. Case material might be presented and students asked to analyze and apply this material based on their newly acquired knowledge. This might either be done through classroom presentations and small-group exercises, or through journaling with specific assignments. Students who are in practice or field settings may be asked to provide examples from their own practice. This type of instruction also introduces supervision.

Finally, ongoing simulations of groups can allow students to participate in situations where they can directly practice their skills and observe others making their own experiments in practice situations. In presenting simulations as an educational option, it is important to add a few caveats. We are not advocating that students participate directly as group members, dealing with their own personal problems. Although exposure to groups as members might be a worthwhile experience, the classroom is not the place for this. Rather, we advocate for a simulation in which members participate within fictionalized characters, either scripted by the instructor or developed by the student, which also helps the student develop "tuning in" skills. We also believe that the group models need to be time limited, with some attention paid to creating a complete group within the classroom. In building in this structure, simulations become more closely aligned with the PBL approach, where students are asked to work through specific problems (e.g., how to implement the model) rather than flounder in unstructured therapeutic situations. This approach also exposes students to all the developmental phases as well as gives them the structure to guide their practice decisions. Finally, the simulation exercise requires time and opportunity to process the activities. This represents a key feature, as the students can use this process to develop their observational skills and integrate classroom information.

In the final stage of the model, instruction moves beyond developing knowledge and practicing skills towards integrating these skills into an articulated whole. This can be accomplished either as an independent set of activities, or as part of the latter stages of experiential exercises. For example, as we detailed in the dynamic model, students need to deal with multiple levels of information and input in responding to practice situation. In the simulation, this would include using critical thinking to integrate theory and models and evidence, the experience in the simulation as it has proceeded over time, and the observations of the group processes as they pertain directly to the situation at hand. Thus, the reflective practitioner emerges out of the ability to process all these elements and arrive at a hypothesis-driven response.

Key to the development of the reflective practitioner is the ability to practice from some sort of integrated and personal practice approach. It is obvious that all of the elements cannot be considered independently for any given practice situation. Although practice over time can increase the group worker's ability to independently integrate elements, much of the integration must be done in advance. This allows the practitioners an existing heuristic that can be used to allow the practitioner to focus on unique or critical elements. Creating some sort of integrated practice statement is a key educational task for the ending stage of the instructional process. Requiring this articulation pushes the group work student to define how the elements will fit together. It further provides a basis from which to focus in on the individual statement. To extend a metaphor from the previous work of one of the authors (Pollio, 2006), the practice statement becomes the canvas, the knowledge elements of the dynamic process (theory, model and evidence) the color palette, and the reflective-practice skills (including the EBP skills) the brush out of which the art of the practice situation emerges.

SUMMARY AND CONCLUSION

Developments in EBP have created challenges to teaching group work, an already complex endeavor. Separate threads of theory, evidence, group models, practice situation, and supervision must be woven together into a dynamic pattern that advances traditional teaching models and adds to the effectiveness of group work. We pulled these elements together in two ways. First, we conceptualized EBP within an integrated instructional model that suggests that all areas are essential in education to advancing effective group work practice. Second, we offered a developmental instructional model to deliver these areas, which may be differentially applied based on the level of knowledge, skill, and experience of the learner. With the inexorable advancements in EBP and the burgeoning and increasingly available group-related research evidence, group worker practitioners and educators may find the two models helpful in understanding how the elements fit together in practice and in teaching. Skill in managing and delivering the various elements of the two models in dynamic practice and teaching situations is an important goal for developing reflective group work practitioners and educators.

ACKNOWLEDGMENT

The authors wish to thank their many students who have, over the years, provided invaluable feedback on the right way to teach group work.

REFERENCES

Borduas, F., Gagnon, R., Lacoursiere, Y., & Laprise, R. (2001). The longitudinal case study: From Schön's model to self-directed learning. *Journal of Continuing Education in the Health Professions, 21*(2), 103–109.

Bricout, J., Pollio, D., Edmond, T., & Moore-McBride, A. (2008).Evidence-based macro practice instruction from an evidence-based perspective. *Journal of Evidence-Based Social Work, 5*, 597–621.

Cartwright, D., & Zander, A. F. (Eds.). (1968). *Group dynamics: Research and theory* (3rd ed.). New York: Harper & Row.

Cournoyer, B. R. (2004). *The evidence-based social work (EBSW) skills book.* Boston: Allyn & Bacon.

Forsyth, D. R. (2009). *Group dynamics* (5th ed.). Belmont, CA: Thomson/ Wadsworth.

Howard, M. O., McMillan, C., & Pollio, D. E. (2003). Teaching evidence-based practice: Toward a new paradigm for social work education.*Research on Social Work Practice, 13*(2), 234–259.

Kerlinger, F. N. (1986). *Foundations of behavioral research* (3rd ed.). New York: Holt, Rinehart and Winston.

Levin, B. B. (2001). *Energizing teacher education and professional development with problem-based learning.* Alexandria, VA: Association for Supervision and Curriculum Development.

Macgowan, M. J. (2008). *A guide to evidence-based group work.* New York: Oxford University Press.

Merriam, S. B. (2001). Andragogy and self-directed learning: Pillars of adult learning theory. In S. B. Merriam (Ed.), *The new update on adult learning theory* (pp. 3–14). San Francisco: Jossey-Bass.

Petrocelli, J. V. (2002). Effectiveness of group cognitive-behavioral therapy for general symptomatology: A meta-analysis. *Journal of Specialists in Group Work, 27*(1), 92–115.

Pollio, D. E., Brower, A., & Galinsky, M. J. (2000). Change in groups. In C. Garvin & P. Allen-Meares (Eds.), *Handbook of social work direct practice* (pp. 281–301). Thousand Oaks, CA: Sage.

Pollio, D. E. (2002). The evidence-based group worker. *Social Work with Groups, 25*(4), 57–70.

Pollio D. E. (2006). The art of evidence-based practice. *Research on Social Work Practice, 16*(2), 224–232.

Rose, S. D. (2004). Cognitive-behavioral group work. In C. D. Garvin, L. M. Gutierrez, M. J. Galinsky (Eds.), *Handbook of social work with groups* (pp. 111–135). New York: Guilford.

Schön, D. A. (1983). *The reflective practitioner: How professionals think in action.* New York: Basic Books.

Schön, D. A. (1987). *Educating the reflective practitioner.* San Francisco: Jossey-Bass.

Schipper, F. (1999). Phenomenology and the reflective practitioner. *Management Learning, 30*(4), 473–485.

Sheafor, B. W., & Horejsi, C. R. (2006). *Techniques and guidelines for social work practice* (7th ed.). Boston: Allyn & Bacon.

Straus, S. E., Richardson, W. S., Glasziou, P., & Haynes, R. B. (2005). *Evidence-based medicine: How to practice and teach EBM* (3rd ed.). Edinburgh, UK: Churchill Livingstone.

Yalom, I. D., & Leszcz, M. (2005). *The theory and practice of group psychotherapy* (5th ed.). New York: Basic Books.

Finding and Integrating the Best Available Evidence into the Group Work Field Practicum: Examples and Experiences from MSW Students

MARK J. MACGOWAN

Florida International University, Miami, Florida, USA

*Evidence-based practice has been widely discussed in the litera-
ture, but little has been said about how it is taught in courses on
group work. This article describes how evidence-based group work
(EBGW) has been taught in a master's level course on group work
and includes examples of students' efforts at utilizing EBGW in
their field placements, and their comments about the experience.
Utilizing a four-stage process model of EBGW, students posed a
clinical question, systematically searched for evidence to answer
the question, critically reviewed the evidence, and applied it into
practice. The examples illustrate the stages of EBGW and highlight
the strengths and limitations of the approach. The written comments provide generally positive feedback and some suggestions for
improvement. Ideas to strengthen the experience are presented.*

Although the principles of evidence-based practice (EBP) have been relatively well explicated and are in mainstream textbooks in social work
education, the practices and challenges of real-world implementation have
prevented widespread adoption. Some of the barriers to implementation
include lack of access to user-friendly summaries of research information,
lack of relevant research to address real-world problems, worries about

"cookbook" approaches to helping, and limited time to access information (Edmond, Megivern, Williams, Rochman, & Howard, 2006).

These challenges are even more pronounced in group work. There have been relatively few discussions in the literature about a systematic process of integrating evidence into group work and about the challenges of applying evidence into group work. Only recently have specific discussions appeared in the literature about the application of evidence into group work (Macgowan, 2006a, 2008; Pollio, 2002, 2006).

The foundations of EBP and evidence-based group work (EBGW) have naturally preceded discussions about actual implementation challenges. Further, within social work education, what is taught in the classroom is often disconnected with what students do in the field placement (Edmond et al., 2006; Howard, McMillan, & Pollio, 2003). Thus, although EBGW may be taught, it is not clear if the learning gets implemented and perhaps more importantly how it gets implemented. This article reports the process and product of an effort to teach EBGW in an academic environment in which EBP is not fully integrated throughout the curriculum, including the field. The author reports the framework for the educational experience, the specific assignments that include an application within their field placements, and provide feedback from the students about the learning experience. The author concludes with suggestions about ways to improve the experience.

OVERVIEW OF EBGW AND THE EDUCATIONAL APPROACH

EBGW has been defined as "a process of the judicious and skillful application in group work of the best evidence, based on research merit, impact, and applicability, using evaluation to ensure desired results are achieved" (Macgowan, 2008, p. 3). Detailed elsewhere (Macgowan, 2008), EBGW is operationalized through a sequence of four stages in which group workers (1) formulate an answerable practice question; (2) search for evidence; (3) undertake a critical review of the evidence (with respect to research merit, impact, and applicability), which yields the best available evidence; and (4) apply the evidence with judgment, skill, and concern for relevance and appropriateness for the group, utilizing evaluation to determine if desired outcomes are achieved. The examples in this article illustrate the four stages.

Although the author teaches some of the fundamentals of EBGW using a traditional, passive, didactic approach, the primary method is problem-based/practice-based learning (PBL). PBL uses an active educational approach by involving students in their learning; it "encourages learners to apply critical thinking, problem-solving skills, and content knowledge to real-world problems and issues" (Levin, 2001, p. 1). Thus, students learn the fundamentals of EBGW through the didactic approach and the process of applying the stages of EBGW through PBL. The educational approach draws on recommendations from other EBP teaching models (e.g., Howard et al., 2003; Straus, Richardson, Glasziou, & Haynes, 2005), which are more fully described in Macgowan (2008).

EBGW is incorporated into a foundation-level graduate class in group work theory and practice. The teaching approach incorporates the four EBGW stages through six class sessions, with the material taught alongside other foundation content in group work. The author uses Toseland and Rivas' book (2005) as the main text and Macgowan (2008) as the supplemental text. Thus, EBGW is one part of the educational component in the course, although the principles underlying EBGW, such as critical thinking, are infused throughout the course work. The course is not taught in a curriculum dedicated to teaching EBP, so the foundation material about EBP must be integrated into the course. Figure 1 provides an example of the elements of EBGW and how they fit into the course.

As indicated in Figure 1, various methods are used to teach the four stages of EBGW. An important part of the learning is derived from two written assignments. The first assignment is concerned with a question each

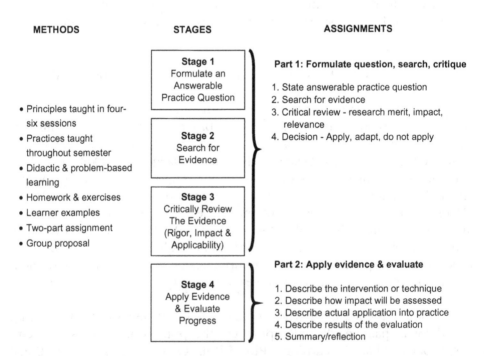

FIGURE 1 Teaching Evidence-Based Group Work in a Foundation Group Work Graduate Course.

Note. Adapted from Macgowan (2008).

student poses about a within-group challenge or problem, such as low verbal participation or low engagement of group members, for which students find, critique, and apply the best available evidence. Any question is appropriate as long as it is a real concern that emerges from a group the student either observes or participates in as a leader or co-leader. This assignment requires students to follow all four stages of EBGW and is divided into two parts, described in the last column of Figure 1. The first part includes the first three stages of EBGW and requires students to formulate a practice-relevant question, search for evidence, critically review the evidence, and decide if/how the evidence would be adapted for the clinical situation. The second part of the assignment requires students to apply the evidence into practice and describe the results of the evaluation. The first example below illustrates this first assignment.

The second assignment is completed by students in groups of five to seven and requires a proposal to develop a treatment group. Students follow the first three stages of EBGW but are not required to implement the proposal. However, they are expected to include in their proposals sufficient detail that it could be readily implemented. As in the first assignment, the process of this assignment begins with a real practice need; students are required to develop a proposal that meets a real need in an agency in the community. The second example below illustrates this assignment.

CASE EXAMPLES

As of this writing, there are no examples in the literature about how EBGW is taught in a group work course. The two examples are from students in an introductory graduate group work course. The field placements were in South Florida and involved groups reflecting the diversity of the area (e.g., proportionately more Latinos and African Americans than Whites). The first example is an effort of a student to manage a within-group challenge in their treatment group. The second example includes two proposals to develop treatment groups, written by two teams of students.

Example 1: Addressing Within-Group Challenges

This assignment requires students to use their groups in their field placements to follow the four stages of EBGW. That is, students are to formulate a practice question related to their group, search for evidence to answer the question, critically evaluate the evidence, and apply it in practice. There are two parts to this assignment due at different times in the semester. The first illustrates the first three stages of EBGW and is due about midsemester. The second part illustrates the fourth stage and is submitted at the end of semester (for a copy of the outline of the assignment, contact the author).

The example cited here is from a student whose field placement was in a community agency in South Florida (Pérez, 2007). She was assigned to work in an existing group consisting of adolescents referred by the courts as part of a diversionary program for first-time offenders. Her role was junior co-leader in the group.

The first stage of EBGW is to formulate a question that comes from the group experience. The student was concerned about two members who rarely participated in the group. She wanted to find a strategy that would help the two integrate more into the group and its activities. An important part of this first step is to critically consider underlying issues that generated the question. The student thoughtfully considered many possible reasons for the lack of involvement. She reviewed the human behavior literature about the functioning of individuals in social situations and explored some literature on shyness and social anxiety. She also considered the group development literature (e.g., Garland, Jones, & Kolodny, 1965) about approach–avoidance conflict noting that "members approach each other in their striving to connect with one another, but they avoid getting too close because they fear the vulnerability that such intimacy implies" (Perez, 2007, p. 2). Thus, the student considered individual and group factors to consider the reasons for the lack of involvement, and to see if any of these factors may provide leads in shaping the question. She concluded that a within-group strategy would be appropriate. The question she formulated was, "In the case of a treatment group for male juvenile first-time offenders who are silent during group activities, what strategy will increase verbal participation?"

Once the question was formulated, the next step was to search the literature for evidence. The first thing to do in this stage is to extract the essential concepts from the question and to formulate keywords to enable a search. In this case, the student identified the following three main concepts: *juvenile offender*, *treatment group*, and *participation*. From these the student developed keywords to form the search string. The keywords for *juvenile offender* were developed by consulting the thesauri of each database searched, which yielded *young offender* and *delinquency*, to name a few. She derived keywords for *treatment group* and *participation* from a list in the author's book (Macgowan, 2008, p. 64). The student recorded the information on a template designed to facilitate searching for evidence (see Macgowan, 2008, p. 76, for a blank copy of the template). As required in the assignment, the student first searched three journal databases (i.e., Social Work Abstracts, Psychological Abstracts, and Educational Resources Information Center [ERIC]), searching the title, keywords, and abstracts, to find if there had been any research studies on the issue or concern (i.e., research evidence). The search yielded no relevant journal articles. Thus, the next step was to find the best authoritative evidence; that is, evidence not explicitly based on formal, rigorous research but on opinion, personal experience, or judgment. Many group work texts are sources for authoritative evidence as they do not usually contain original, peer-reviewed research studies, but rather the authors' perspectives on areas of group work, which may or may not be based on the findings of formal research studies. However, because books may be the only sources for published evidence, albeit authoritative, they are valuable and can become the "best available evidence." In her search of this literature, the student did not find any book specifically in the area she was looking for (i.e., juvenile offenders in groups). Instead, she found a book that included specific strategies for increasing group member's verbal participation (Jacobs, Masson, & Harvill, 1998). She explained that the most appropriate strategy to use was drawing out through the use of rounds:

> Drawing out is the term used by Jacobs and colleagues (1998) to refer to the skill of eliciting group members' comments. Getting members to go deeper is a form of drawing out that is very helpful to members in support, growth, counseling, and therapy groups (Jacobs et al., 1998, p. 162). A way to draw out members is through the use of rounds.
>
> With the use of rounds, the leader asks everyone to comment without singling out any one member. There are three kinds of rounds: (1) the designated word/phrase or number round, (2) the word or phrase round, and (3) the comment round (Jacobs et al., 1998). The kind of round to be used to get the above-mentioned adolescents to participate more in group activities will be the comment round. This type of round is used when the leader wants members to say more than just a few words. In addition, since the members have to say comments instead of just words or phrases, the member has more control over the content and length of time, and everyone gets a chance to speak what is on their mind. In the present situation being discussed, the intention is to get these two members to share more. Therefore, two separate rounds will be used and on each one the round will end in one of the two individuals that are to be drawn out, so the leader will be able to focus more on what those two members have to say, and perhaps more easily ask the members to elaborate on their comment, since they will be the last ones to speak. (Pérez, 2007, p. 2,9)

The third stage is to evaluate critically the evidence in the areas of rigor, impact, and applicability using an appropriate guide. Using the guide to evaluate the quality of authority-based evidence (Macgowan, 2008, pp. 142–144), the student rated the rigor and impact of the source (i.e., Jacobs et al., 1998) as strong. An important consideration in determining the applicability of a technique or an intervention is cultural applicability, particularly in locations such as Miami-Dade County in South Florida. Much of the evidence about group work has been developed using dominant racial/cultural groups.

Multicultural competence is important in EBP (Chen, Kakkad, & Balzano, 2008) and essential in settings that serve diverse groups. In this example, the student concluded that applicability was high. There was nothing significant that prevented her from applying the technique in the multicultural field setting in which she was placed. The only caveat she noted was that she would follow the recommendation of the authors (Jacobs et al., 1998) who recommended that with adolescents, the technique of drawing out group members should be used delicately, giving the members the opportunity to speak while also giving them the opportunity to decline. Thus, the student concluded that the technique found was sufficiently rigorous, impactful, and applicable to use in the group.

The fourth stage is to apply the technique. Here is how the student described how she was going to use the technique to encourage the two group members to participate verbally:

> First, I intend to place the members in a circle, as the current setting of the group is more of a U-shape, with the leader's chair in the open part of the *U*-shape. Second, I will propose the question to be used in the first round. The question to be used in this round will be: "When you think of the choice you had to either come to [the agency] or go to court to have your case tried, what feelings or thoughts did you have? Take a moment to think about this and then we'll do a round." If needed, I will give an example of the type of answer they can provide, such as: "I'm glad I chose [this agency] because at least I won't be sent to jail." I will begin this round with the person closest to member A [one of the silent youths] and will go around the room until I finish with him. I will then attempt to expand on what he says. I will ask him additional questions to invite him to open up about his feelings of being at [the agency]. Once this has been done, I will address any feelings this round may have surfaced in the members, and then I will begin a second round, this time beginning with the person nearest group member B [the other silent group member]. The question to be used in this round will be: "Knowing the consequences of going to jail, and with the information you have learned at this agency so far, what actions do you plan to take so you don't get in trouble with the law again? We're going to do a round to hear from everyone." Again, I will finish the round with member B, and focus on his answers to expand and get him to speak more about his plans, thoughts, and feelings. (Pérez, 2007, p. 3–4)

To evaluate the effects of the technique, the student reported that she would use a single-subject design (SSD), specifically, an A-B design. The student offered the following details:

> This type of SSD requires the repeated measurement of some behavior during the baseline (A phase) and also during the intervention (B) phase. The baseline will be drawn retrospectively, counting the previous three

meeting sessions and then tallying the number of verbal contributions in the following three sessions after the use of the comment rounds. Verbal contributions to be tallied will be complete sentences, whether in response to open-ended questions or as contribution to the topic of discussion. Simple utterances or answers to close-ended questions will not be included in the tally. (Pérez, 2007, p. 5)

The student's goal was to have the two members participate in group sessions more than twice per session. To record this, she used a chart to record the frequency of member communication in group sessions derived from the main textbook used in the course (Toseland & Rivas, 2005, p. 240). The student reported that she was nervous implementing the technique, largely because it was the first session in which she took the lead in the session, although she was present in earlier sessions and occasionally contributed. She reported that the group members contributed more after the implementation of the technique. Member A continued to contribute in the subsequent sessions, noticeably more than during baseline. Member B also increased his contributions, but at a lesser level.

To improve the intervention, the student recommended that comment rounds be used in an earlier stage of group development, and throughout the life of the group. She also recommended that it would be helpful if a co-worker tally the verbal contributions: "Counting the number of verbal participations, whether they may be words or complete sentences, can get too cumbersome for the group leader, as it did for me" (Pérez, 2007, p. 8).

In concluding the assignment, the student made the following comment about the experience:

I had never been exposed to group work until this semester and I do not know a lot about effective techniques to implement in groups. However, Jacobs et al., (1998) stated that "no skill, technique, or exercise is more valuable that the use of rounds" (p. 175). . . . Therefore, this intervention should be used in groups where there are silent group members, but it should be planned more carefully to ensure an effective and efficient implementation. Using an evidence-based group approach, although somewhat tedious given the amount of work that needs to be done prior to determining which intervention to use with a specific group, gives more credibility to the group leader. An evidence-based intervention carries the influence of previous researchers and group workers who have tested its rigor, applicability, and impact and have concluded that the intervention is effective. Conducting evidence-based research is not a simple or quick task, but I have learned that it is worthwhile if the group leader wishes to be successful when implementing an intervention within a group. For this reason, it is very gratifying to have learned about group work, ways to conduct groups, and ways to gather evidence on a specific intervention I may be interested in implementing in the future. (Pérez, 2007, p. 9)

This first example illustrated the four stages of EBGW. Some important points should be highlighted from the perspective of the learner and educator. First, the example highlights how everyday practice dilemmas (e.g., silent members) may not be answered by research evidence. EBGW requires group workers to use the best available evidence, which may not have been formally researched but instead based on an author's recommendation. This challenges some notions of EBP that suggest that only research evidence is valid. Although research-based evidence is generally preferred because rigorous research studies reduce potential biases that plague authority-based evidence (Gambrill, 1999), relatively few group work practices and models have been tested in empirical research. Thus, EBGW may include authority-based evidence if that is the only evidence available after undergoing the vetting process. The term *best available evidence* is used to indicate that the evidence has been vetted through the first three stages of EBGW, which may yield, preferably, research-based evidence, but also authority-based evidence.

Second, engaging in EBGW for the first time is tedious! Much time is spent formulating a practice question, finding, evaluating, and applying into practice the best available evidence. Everything occurs in slow motion, which is a by-product of learning new critical skills. Here are a couple of e-mails the author received after the students' initial foray into searching the literature:

- Dear Prof. Macgowan. Good afternoon. I know last week you said we would be lucky to find at least three articles on our topic, but I am encountering even worse difficulties. Everything I find that is even remotely similar to my keywords/concepts, there are only abstracts for them or I have to pay crazy amounts of money to be able to download the entire article. Is this to be expected, or am I doing something completely wrong? I appreciate any feedback you can provide.
- Professor Macgowan. I have never had this much difficulty searching for an article in my life. It is very frustrating. The articles that I found that would come close to the topic I have, charges a particular fee to get a copy. I printed out a couple of articles but after reading them I don't think they will be helpful. I am really at a loss for words. What can I do now?

The students' messages were used as the basis for class discussion and resolution. The first message, not readily finding material, is often resolved by expanding the search by removing concepts and/or by moving beyond from searching only for journals to searching for books. The second issue, not finding material at no cost, is sometimes resolved by using interlibrary loan, if there is time. If they cannot be acquired in time, the materials are considered not available and students are instructed to move on to find other material (for readers without access to a university's online materials, a number of resources are available at no cost at www.EvidenceBasedGroupWork.com). In the author's experience over the past several years, these two concerns have been resolved through class discussion. However, this raises a third issue. Educators have to be flexible and willing to use examples drawn from student's struggles. This is a departure from traditional learning approaches that use lectures and canned examples. In case-based learning, educators have to be prepared to (1) manage students' (and their own) frustrations at the lack of high-quality research evidence, (2) invite the rest of the class to help in the process of resolution, and (3) be flexible in helping students resolve within-group challenges to a reasonable but not perfect resolution. Finding the best available evidence for dealing with real practice concerns takes critical thinking, patience, flexibility, and resourcefulness.

Example 2: Developing a Proposal to Establish a Group to Address a Community Concern

The main purpose of the second assignment is for students to develop skill in developing a research-based proposal for a group service that addresses a real concern in a local agency in Miami-Dade County. The proposal assignment differs from the first assignment in three ways. First, students only complete the first three stages of EBGW. Second, students are required to find a higher level of evidence; namely, high-quality research evidence supporting the efficacy of the proposed group intervention. The group intervention must have been tested in rigorous research and demonstrated to be effective in reducing problems or risk factors, or in strengthening protective factors. Because this assignment is limited to group interventions with good research support, it excludes a number of possibly helpful group approaches. However, the point of the assignment is to deliver a proposal for a group service with demonstrably effective results. The third way in which this assignment differs from the first is the topic (or question) is derived from a host agency in the community. The author developed an informal partnership with a large substance abuse and mental health treatment center to identify pressing needs that a group service may address. At the beginning of the semester, a representative of the agency visited the class to discuss the needs facing clients in the agency. The needs became the questions the students used to develop a group proposal. At the end of the semester, students presented their papers to the agency representative. This partnership is an exciting opportunity for students to have a real impact in the community. In addition, many agencies would like to implement evidence-based practices but lack the staff or time to do it on their own, so this partnership is a good opportunity for them.

Two proposals are described, along with how they developed over the first three stages of EBGW (for a copy of the outline of the assignment, contact the author).

To begin the first stage of EBGW, the agency representative came to class and described a number of needs. One that was presented was the need for a group to reduce sexually transmitted diseases (STDs) among adolescents with substance abuse problems. STDs were becoming more prevalent among adolescents seeking services at the center. A second need was for a proposal that would include a "stages of change" approach for the reduction in substance abuse for adults. The stages of change model (Connors, Donovan, & DiClemente, 2001) has been widely discussed in the literature, but relatively understudied in groups. The agency representative wanted to know if there was a research-based model for adults. Thus, two student groups were formed that formulated two questions. The first question was, "In the case of a group of adolescents with alcohol and other drug problems, what group intervention is the most effective in reducing the risk of STDs?" (Benavides, Chirito, Drzewicki, & Bilderbeek, 2008, p. 2). The second question was, "In the case of adults with substance abuse problems, how can the stages of change model be implemented in group work?" (Levy, Peña, Sanchez, & Thomas, 2008, p. 3).

The search for evidence was similar to the process in the first assignment, but broader. In addition to searching within three journal databases, students were required to search in sites that included systematic reviews, such as Cochrane Collaboration or Campbell Collaboration (see Macgowan, 2008, pp. 46–48, for other examples and Websites). The assignment required at least one research study that was rigorous and impactful. In addition, the assignment required that the group intervention must be well described, such as in a treatment manual (for a discussion about the function of manuals in EBP, see Galinsky, Terzian, & Fraser, 2006; Macgowan, 2008, p. 112). In the first example (group for adolescents at risk for STDs), students found a few group-based interventions, which lacked sufficient detail about the groups. The one that the students finally selected included a manual available online (Rotheram-Borus et al., 2001). In the second example (stages of change), students found an authoritative source describing a relevant intervention. Normally, this would not fulfill the expectations of the assignment, which required research evidence. However, the students contacted the author of the authoritative source, who sent the students a scholarly conference paper that included findings from a randomized clinical trial that tested the stages of change model in group therapy for adults who abused cocaine. This fulfilled the general expectations of the assignment (i.e., research evidence, manualized).

At the third stage of EBGW, both student teams critically evaluated the quality of the evidence using a guide. In the first case (group for adolescents at risk for STDs), students used the guide for evaluating a randomized clinical trial (Macgowan, 2008, pp. 104–109) and rated the rigor as moderate and impact as strong (i.e., the intervention appeared to make good improvement among group members). The group intervention was judged to be applicable to the situation and for the group members intended. In the second case (stages of change), students used the guide to evaluate a randomized clinical trial and rated the rigor of the study as moderate to strong. They rated impact as strong, as there was good clinical evidence of change among group members. The students thought the group intervention was applicable to the proposed setting and population. Thus, in both cases, students believed that the evidence they found was sufficiently rigorous, impactful, and applicable that they would propose these group models.

Although students were not required to enter into the fourth stage of EBGW, students were required to prepare for it. They were required to identify (1) if and how the intervention may need to be adapted to make it more applicable, (2) a research design to evaluate the effectiveness of the intervention, (3) reliable and valid outcome measures so that change could be measured, and (4) a measure of group process, such as the Group Engagement Measure (Macgowan, 2006b). Students also included information about leadership, timing, membership, physical environment, recruitment, a general budget, discussion about anticipated problems, and an advertisement for the group.

At the end of the semester, each group made a brief presentation of the proposal to the class and to the representative of the agency. This is an important time for the students to share thoughts about the process and for the representative to ask questions.

STUDENTS' COMMENTS ABOUT THE ASSIGNMENTS

For two semesters over 2007 and 2008, students provided written comments about their experiences with the two EBGW assignments, after final grades were assigned. Five questions were asked, four open-ended and one closed-ended. Out of a total of 37 possible responses, 7 were received, representing a sample of 19%. There were six females and one male, five white Latinos(as), one White non-Latino(a), and one Asian American. The sections below provide the questions asked, students' responses, and the author's commentary.

What Did You Learn From the Assignment? What Was Beneficial About the Assignment?

One student reflected on how she learned how to identify and conceptualize a group concern and search for relevant research.

In both the individual and large group assignment, I learned how to identify a problem/concern at my agency. In addition, I learned how to operationalize the problem/concern and develop the question. The question facilitated the search for relevant research to address the problem.

Other students reported that the assignments helped them learn how to search and critique material obtained from the search. However, the biggest comment from all students was that they benefitted specifically from learning how to critically evaluate group-related research.

- I learned a lot from both assignments but the one that I really learned the most from was the [first assignment]. From the assignment I learned how to efficiently search for articles and define my search of articles. I learned how to narrow down my searches in the different library databases. The assignment taught me how to focus my search and writing when working with groups. The assignment allowed me to read articles in different areas and learn to pick the best article available. The appraisal process of the assignment allowed me to look at things in articles that normally I would not look at and analyze.
- The most beneficial part of the assignment was learning how to critically evaluate research. As social workers, we cannot automatically assume that research that has been published is quality research. Both assignments provided us with the tools necessary to be able to identify flaws and/or biases in published research. The guides provided by the instructor gave us a road map as to what areas to focus on.
- I learned how to critically analyze research articles. As students/practitioners, we're bombarded with research articles on every subject. It is a bit overwhelming trying to figure out which one has demonstrated soundness in research methods and which article is weak. This assignment taught me to distinguish between articles and choose the ones that are grounded in sound research methods.
- I believe that this assignment allowed me to properly evaluate the strength of a research article. Prior to this, I was unsure as to precisely what criteria constituted strong research. This assignment was also beneficial because it allowed me to perform an actual trial run of an evidence-based group intervention and see how well it worked in practice. [first assignment]
- I have taken no other course in which the process of analyzing a research report was so completely laid out.

How Do You Think the Assignments Have Helped You as a Group Worker?

Students reported that the assignments helped them become aware of the range of possible group interventions. One student wrote, "I became more aware of the extent of research on working with groups." Students also reported that they became more attuned to group process and how to find group-based research.

- Both assignments made me more cognizant of group processes. In the individual assignment [first assignment], my agency was having difficulty recruiting members to our support groups. The assignment broadened my knowledge about possible barriers that would discourage attendance and different methods to improve them. Furthermore, both assignments provided me with a clear and simple way to search for group specific research that in turn will help to enhance my group work skills.
- As the assignment was to choose a research article that is group based, it discussed group processes. This was particularly helpful as I learned the different ways of increasing group engagement and developing group processes. In the future, this assignment will aid me in choosing group-related research that fits with what I want to do in my group. At my internship, when trying to decide how to conduct my anger management group, I was able to filter through several group-related research articles and find the ones that had good rigor, impact, and applicability to the situation. This was possible as a result of this assignment.
- The assignment allowed me to focus my search to group work, instead of looking at articles and research that focused on the individual. The assignment allowed me to understand the group process and dynamics better. The assignment allowed me to read about different types of groups and to read about the [types of] research done on groups.

Another student reported that she learned more about evaluating group work:

> I think this assignment demonstrated to me how to evaluate whether or not the group intervention was working effectively while the group was still ongoing. This allowed me to assess more rapidly whether or not I needed to move on to another technique.

How Would You Improve the Assignment?

One student lamented that she could not see the group proposal implemented: "It would have been beneficial to have implemented the intervention or method in our agency setting. This would have provided us with the opportunity to experience the entire process from developing a research question to carrying out the proposed technique."

The next comment reflects a limitation of some of our field placements that lack either groups or experienced group workers for supervision. If a student is without a group work experience, he or she works with another student and they do the assignment together.

I cannot think of any improvements that could be made to the actual assignment. However, some of my classmates were unable to work first hand with a group at his or her internship due to the types of programs run in his or her placement agency. I believe that being directly involved in the implementation of the research was a valuable lesson that some of my classmates may have missed out on, even though these individuals were allowed to partner up with others who were involved with a group at his or her placement agency.

One student identified an issue that has become an essential class discussion topic. Students need help in deciding what to do with evidence that did not readily fit after the search for evidence was completed. The student noted that,

Despite encouragement that I would find what I first wanted to study, I finally came to the conclusion that research on my intended topic did not exist. I wound up changing my topic because I found other articles that discussed a different but related problem. I recognize that it is difficult to keep track of all the different subjects being explored within a class, but I felt there was not enough allowance for helping students recognize signs of a dead end.

The author encouraged the student to keep the original question, as it represented a real practice problem, but instead pursue a systematic process of widening the search criteria by dropping less relevant concepts/key words from the search strategy and by expanding into authority-based evidence. This approach validated the original question and the important function of authority-based evidence in EBGW.

Please Provide Any Other Comments About the Learning Experience

One student responded that they appreciated the structured, systematic approach to finding evidence: "Your organization and step-by-step guides to analysis are very useful to the student. I felt that I was learning a logical, replicable process and was relying less on brute effort and luck." Students valued the skills in evaluating research. One student noted, "I found the skills I learned in evaluating research will be ones that I use over and over again as I pursue a research career. Thank you for giving me the building blocks to start with!" Another student noted, "Your input and guidance were invaluable. The *Guide to Evidence-Based Group Work* is definitely a tool to learn all the 'how-tos' in preparing for research and serves as a reference manual for future research projects." Other students added the following comments:

- Overall, I believe that this assignment has given me more practical knowledge and experience than any other assignment I have completed in my Master's program. I finally feel like I have a good grasp on how to critically appraise and implement an intervention.
- I believe this assignment will benefit me not only in evaluating group-related research, but evaluating research in general. Because the assignment provided guidelines to analyze research articles, it makes it easy to determine what research to use and what to avoid. Prior to this class, no guidelines were offered in regards to critically analyzing research articles. These guidelines have provided me with a frame of reference so that I can do a mental check every time I read a research article to determine its rigor, impact, and applicability. Clearly, this is a skill every student should develop in graduate school in order to provide clinical services grounded in evidenced based practices.
- The course was overall a really good class. I learned a lot from the class that I am applying actually to my classes right now. I learned a lot of things that I know I could and will apply to my work once I start working in the field. The professor provided a comfortable and fun learning environment.

As Result of Completing the Assignment, How Much Did You Learn About Finding and Critically Evaluating Group-Related Research? (1 = *very little*; 2 = *little*; 3 = *some*; 4 = *much*; 5 = *very much*)

Six of the seven students reported *very much* and one student reported *much*. The student who reported *much* added the following comment: "Nearly all of my courses at [Florida International University] have been strongly oriented toward finding and critically evaluating appropriate empirical research. Yours has been as good as any of the other courses, probably better."

These data represent a small sample of possible respondents and represent satisfied consumers. The responses were not anonymous, although they were submitted after grades were assigned. To determine if these data reflect the opinions of just the few who responded, the author reviewed the university's anonymous quantitative and qualitative course evaluations for the same time period ($n = 27$, 73% of respondents). Although the numerical ratings do not ask about specific assignments, the global ratings of satisfaction of the course were very favorable (ratings for summer and fall, 2007 and fall 2008 are available from: http://w3.fiu.edu/irdata/portal/instructor_eval.asp). The few qualitative comments received were also positive.

SUMMARY, RECOMMENDATIONS, AND CONCLUSIONS

This article described the author's approach in educating master's level students about EBGW. Students reported that they benefitted from the experience. Although the comments were favorable, the effect of the learning on actual practice is unknown. An important next step is to assess how students use EBGW in their subsequent field placements and after graduation.

This article presented one method of teaching EBGW. The approach is evolving, and a few comments can be made about how the experience may be improved in our setting. First, the basic principles of EBP should be taught in the first year of the curriculum. Indeed, for EBGW to be more effective, it needs to be infused throughout the curriculum (Walker, Briggs, Koroloff, & Friesen, 2007). The course described in this article is taught in the first semester of the second year and is the only one in the curriculum to include the stages of EBP. No previous course introduces the concepts of EBP, such as critical thinking, formulating a question, and searching for and evaluating evidence (i.e., information literacy). Such content should be covered in an earlier course, which would allow the group work course to emphasize adaptations for group work.

Second, field advisors and group work supervisors should be trained in EBGW. None of the students in this article had advisors or supervisors who were trained in the principles of EBGW, which is a testament to the student's knowledge and skill in working independently. Students were often teaching their supervisors about principles of EBGW. The learning experience would be greatly enhanced with advisors who could engage students within the field setting about how evidence may be implemented, and students could involve their supervisors in the process of evaluating evidence to determine applicability. Without the field advisor and supervisor as an educational partner, EBGW cannot fully develop.

Although coordination within the curriculum is important, better success may be achieved with coordination at higher levels of systems such as the school and agency level, involving agency leadership to the line worker, and even larger systems involving accrediting bodies (Proctor, 2007). This strategy would involve the creation of an EBGW task force involving curriculum representatives, local service providers, and representatives from the local chapters of the Association for the Advancement of Social Work with Groups. A number of other solutions to the challenges of teaching EBP are described in special issues of *Research on Social Work Practice* (September 2007) and *Journal of Social Work Education* (Fall 2007).

In conclusion, teaching EBGW requires flexibility, perseverance, and grace, from educators and students. However, what is gained from the process are knowledge and critical skills for finding the best available evidence for improving the helpfulness of group work. From their comments, students reported that the process was worthwhile and that their critical thinking skills about group work were developed. There is much to be done to improve the teaching of EBGW, and to advance the demonstrable effectiveness of social work with groups we should commit to the process of working together to develop solutions.

ACKNOWLEDGMENT

Acknowledgements to the following students whose examples and/or comments are included in this report: Delimar Pérez, Maribel Benavides, Fiorella Chirito, Lauren Drzewicki, Angela van Bilderbeek, Lourdes Levy, Christine Peña, Naida Sanchez, Latrice Thomas, Lisbeth Fernandez, Pamela Gormley, Amber Jeansonne, Jenna Kramer, Leah Warden, Ramon Bello, Lindsay Brown, and Bisma Sayed.

REFERENCES

Benavides, M., Chirito, F., Drzewicki, L., & Bilderbeek, A. v. (2008). *Together learning choices: An evidence-based group intervention for reducing risk for sexually transmitted diseases*. Unpublished manuscript, School of Social Work, Florida International University, Miami.

Chen, E. C., Kakkad, D., & Balzano, J. (2008). Multicultural competence and evidence-based practice in group therapy. *Journal of Clinical Psychology*, *64*(11), 1261–1278.

Connors, G. J., Donovan, D. M., & DiClemente, C. C. (2001). *Substance abuse treatment and the stages of change: Selecting and planning interventions*. New York: Guilford Press.

Edmond, T., Megivern, D., Williams, C., Rochman, E., & Howard, M. (2006). Integrating evidence-based practice and social work field education. *Journal of Social Work Education*, *42*(2), 377–396.

Galinsky, M. J., Terzian, M. A., & Fraser, M. W. (2006). The art of group work practice with manualized curricula. *Social Work with Groups*, *29*(1), 11–26.

Gambrill, E. (1999). Evidence-based clinical practice: An alternative to authority-based practice. *Families in Society*, *80*, 341–350.

Garland, J. A., Jones, H. E., & Kolodny, R. L. (1965). A model for stages of development in social work groups. In S. Bernstein (Ed.), *Explorations in group work: Essays in theory and practice* (pp. 12–53). Boston: Boston University School of Social Work.

Howard, M. O., McMillan, C. J., & Pollio, D. E. (2003). Teaching evidence-based practice: Toward a new paradigm for social work education. *Research on Social Work Practice*, *13*(2), 234–259.

Jacobs, E. E., Masson, R. L., & Harvill, R. L. (1998). *Group counseling: Strategies and skills* (3rd ed.). Pacific Grove, CA: Brooks/Cole.

Levin, B. B. (2001). *Energizing teacher education and professional development with problem-based learning*. Alexandria, VA: Association for Supervision and Curriculum Development.

Levy, L., Peña, C., Sanchez, N., & Thomas, L. (2008). *Group proposal: Stages of change in groups*. Unpublished manuscript, School of Social Work, Florida International University, Miami.

Macgowan, M. J. (2006a). Evidence-based group work: A framework for advancing best practice. *Journal of Evidence-Based Social Work*, *3*(1), 1–21.

Macgowan, M. J. (2006b). The Group Engagement Measure: A review of its conceptual and empirical properties. *Journal of Groups in Addiction and Recovery*, *1*(2), 33–52.

Macgowan, M. J. (2008). *A guide to evidence-based group work*. New York: Oxford University Press.

Pérez, D. (2007). *Increasing verbal participation of silent group members*. Unpublished manuscript, School of Social Work, Florida International University, Miami.

Pollio, D. E. (2002). The evidence-based group worker. *Social Work with Groups*, *25*(4), 57–70.

Pollio, D. E. (2006). The art of evidence-based practice. *Research on Social Work Practice*, *16*(2), 224–232.

Proctor, E. K. (2007). Implementing evidence-based practice in social work education: Principles, strategies, and partnerships. *Research on Social Work Practice*, *17*(5), 583–591.

Rotheram-Borus, M. J., Lee, M. B., Murphy, D. A., Futterman, D., Duan, N., Birnbaum, J. M., et al. (2001). Efficacy of a preventive intervention for youths living with HIV. *American Journal of Public Health*, *91*(3), 400–405.

Straus, S. E., Richardson, W. S., Glasziou, P., & Haynes, R. B. (2005). *Evidence-based medicine: How to practice and teach EBM* (3rd ed.). Edinburgh, UK: Churchill Livingstone.

Toseland, R. W., & Rivas, R. F. (2005). *An introduction to group work practice* (5th ed.). Boston: Pearson/Allyn and Bacon.

Walker, J. S., Briggs, H. E., Koroloff, N., & Friesen, B. J. (2007). Implementing and sustaining evidence-based practice in social work. *Journal of Social Work Education*, *43*(3), 361–375.

"We may not like it but we guess we have to do it:" Bringing Agency-Based Staff on Board with Evidence-Based Group Work

BARBARA MUSKAT

The Hospital for Sick Children, Toronto, Ontario, Canada

FAYE MISHNA, FATANEH FARNIA, and JUDITH WIENER

University of Toronto, Toronto, Ontario, Canada

In this article the authors describe our experience of developing a manualized model of group treatment for early adolescents with learning disabilities. We review the process of developing and piloting the manual as part of a school-based intervention research project, and the process and complexities in using this model in a community agency with a long history of conducting groups. The authors provide the leaders' feedback on their experience of co-leading a manualized group approach. They conclude with practice principles and recommendations based on the staff's feedback, with respect to bringing agency-based workers on board with an evidence-based approach to group work practice.

INTRODUCTION

The growing demand for evidence-based practice (EBP) presents a healthy challenge for group work practitioners (Macgowan, 2006; Pollio, 2002). To undertake this challenge, practitioners have begun to develop, pilot, evaluate, and disseminate group work models that demonstrate effectiveness. Dissemination of effective models of group work allows these to be further piloted and modified for diverse audiences. Treatment manuals typically comprise descriptions of the group purpose and content, targeted participants, and implementation procedures. The manualization of group work models enhances the likelihood of fidelity and accurate replication (Galinsky, Terzian, & Fraser, 2006).

Along with a significant increase in the number of manualized group models, the use of manualized curricula in groups is growing and is seen as an asset (Comer, Meier, & Galinsky, 2004). Nevertheless, there are well-documented critiques of treatment manuals (Carroll & Nuro, 2002; Galinsky et al., 2006; McMurran & Duggan, 2005). These include beliefs that manuals are overly focused on content to the exclusion of process, are overly prescriptive and do not consider the needs of individual members, and are not tailored to diverse populations (Carroll & Nuro, 2002; Chorpita, 2002; Kurland & Salmon, 2002; Westen, Novotny, & Thompson-Brenner, 2004).

In this article we describe our experience of developing a manualized model of group treatment for early adolescents with learning disabilities (LDs). We review the process of developing and piloting the manual as part of a school-based intervention research project, and the process and complexities in using this model in a community agency with a long history of conducting groups. We provide the leaders' feedback on their experience of co-leading a manualized group approach. We conclude with practice principles and recommendations based on the staff's feedback, with respect to bringing agency-based workers on board with an evidence-based approach to group work practice.

CHALLENGES FOR GROUP WORKERS

Present-day social workers who deliver group services face a number of challenges. First, with a renewed demand for generic practitioners who are expected to be competent in a broad range of practice and research, social workers must develop and maintain skills in a number of modalities, such as practice with individuals, couples, and families, advocacy, evaluation, and group. This increasing demand is coupled with a decline in the teaching of group work practice in social work programs (Goodman & Muniz, 2004; Kurland et al., 2004; McNicoll & Lindsay, 2002).

A second challenge that goes along with the need to attain multiple skills is the advent of managed care in a time of shrinking resources (Kurland & Salmon, 2002; Kurland et al., 2004). One result is the need for practitioners to "do more with less," as quickly and cheaply as possible. Group work is considered less expensive (McDermott, 2003) and at least as beneficial as individual psychotherapy (Burlingame & Krogel, 2005).

A third challenge in social work and other fields is the important and increasing focus on EBP. According to Pollio (2006), EBP includes the "conscientious and judicious use of current best practice in making decisions for individual treatment" (p. 225). EBP has also been described as "the intersection of current best external evidence, client values and expectations, and practitioner expertise" (Shlonsky & Gibbs, 2004). EBP demonstrates the value, quality, and effectiveness of service (Mace, 2006).

Over the past number of years there has been a greater amount of research conducted on the effectiveness of group intervention (Ward, 2004). Despite cautions about the potential for harm in groups (Galinsky & Schopler, 1977; Roback, 2000), there is evidence that "groups work" (Barlow, Burlingame, & Fuhriman, 2000; Burlingame, Fuhriman, & Mosier, 2003; Hoag & Burlingame, 1997). Group work benefits individuals across the life span (Bratton, Ray, Rhine, & Jones, 2005; Hoag & Burlingame, 1997; Page, Weiss, & Lietaer, 2001; Weisz, Weiss, Han, Granger, & Morton, 1995), including children and adolescents (Cramer-Azima, 2002).

In a meta-analysis of group treatment with children and adolescents, Hoag and Burlingame (1997) examined 56 outcome studies and found that the average child or youth in group treatment is better off than 73% of those in control groups. Kulic, Horne, and Dagley (2004) examined 94 studies of prevention groups for children and adolescents and discovered that though studies demonstrated effectiveness, many did not have adequate descriptions of their intervention procedures, thus limiting the opportunity for other clinicians to use the models in practice. The authors asserted, "we are past the point where we can simply say that 'groups work' ... and omit details of how they work" (p. 143) and commented that the lack of detail makes the findings of little clinical or practical value. Kulic and colleagues further proposed that research in group work must include explication of intervention procedures, preferably through the development of treatment manuals. According to the authors, the use of manuals prevents the delivery of group interventions based on inaccurate interpretations of poorly described procedures.

EVIDENCE-BASED PRACTICE

The Code of Ethics of the National Association of Social Workers, the Practice Statement of the Canadian Association of Social Workers, and the *Standards for Social Work Practice with Groups* emphasize the importance of basing practice on recognized knowledge, maintaining currency with emerging knowledge, promoting evaluation and research that contributes to the development of new knowledge, and disseminating knowledge of effective practices relevant to social work (Association for the Advancement of Social Work with Groups, 2005; Canadian Association of Social Workers

[CASW], 2000; National Association of Social Workers [NASW], 1999). These statements are congruent with the principles of EBP described above.

Evidence-based group work comprises appraising systematically, collected evidence from a variety of sources, evaluating the outcomes of practice, implementing models of practice consistently, attending to individual differences in practice decisions and incorporating evidence in understanding group process, leadership, and development (Macgowan, 2006; Pollio, 2002). Practitioners who subscribe to evidence-based group work must maintain currency about research, learn about new models, carefully consider the rationale for treatment decisions, evaluate their own practice, and report findings from their experiences in group work practice journals (Pollio, 2002). This clearly requires the commitment of considerable time and resources by practitioners and sponsoring agencies, ideally including time and resources to design interventions, supervision on group leadership, and consultation on evaluation procedures. With today's limited resources, the commitment to EBP may be present, whereas the resources may not.

Although many group work practitioners may be current with respect to evidence-based approaches to research and evaluation, they do not necessarily employ them (Brower, Arndt, & Ketterhagen, 2004). Difficulties that group workers associate with evaluation and research include ethical problems related to randomly assigning and withholding treatment from control groups in random controlled studies, the small number of participants in groups that do not achieve statistical power, adherence to treatment methods that do not meet the unique needs of group members, and methods that fail to capture the "groupness" of groups.

TREATMENT MANUALS

Treatment manuals are guides to the application of therapeutic procedures. A well-designed treatment manual describes treatment strategies and the ways to apply them in a specific approach (McMurran & Duggan, 2005). Included are details about the theoretical framework, the model of intervention, and implementation guidelines.

There is growing recognition of the importance of treatment manuals in evidence-based intervention (Galinsky et al., 2006; Scaturo, 2001). Advantages of manuals include their explication of treatment models and their underlying theories. Manuals encourage adherence to a treatment model, thus increasing integrity. Manuals assist training of experienced group workers in new models and contribute to the development of less experienced staff (Carroll & Nuro, 2002; McMurran & Duggan, 2005). Manuals permit clinicians to follow a prescribed sequence of events that can be replicated by others (Kendall, Chu, Gifford, Hayes, & Nauta, 1998).

Finally, manuals foster comparisons among treatment approaches and permit multiple treatment trials, which leads to refinement of treatment approaches. Thus, treatment manuals are major contributors to the development of a collection of evidence-based resources.

A number of disadvantages to the use of manuals have been identified. A great deal has been written about clinicians' reluctance to adopt manualized programs (Addis & Krasnow, 2000; Beutler, 2002; Carroll & Nuro, 2002; Kendall et al., 1998; Kurland & Salmon, 2002; McMurran & Duggan, 2005). Other critiques include the lack of applicability to complex client populations and attention to group dynamics and treatment alliances (Carroll & Nuro, 2002; Kurland & Salmon, 2002), the overly restrictive structure and lack of room for clinical judgment and flexibility (Kendall et al., 1998; McMurran & Duggan, 2005), and for the development of mutual aid (Kurland & Salmon, 2002). Further, manualized programs are depicted as offering a "one-size-fits-all" approach to treatment, therefore not meeting the specific needs of individual clients (Beutler, 2002) or of diverse groups (Chorpita, 2002). Some practitioners view manuals as driven by managed care and catering to approaches that "do more with less" in response to diminished resources (Kurland & Salmon, 2002). Others consider manuals as cookbooks that lack the cook's creativity (Kendall et al., 1998, p. 178), and as diminishing the "art" of therapy (Galinsky et al., 2006).

Research that examines therapists' views of manuals has yielded mixed results. Addis and Krasnow (2000) conducted a survey on practitioners' attitudes and beliefs about treatment manuals. One third of the respondents were not clear what a treatment manual was, and 40% had never used one. Although many of the practitioners had given very little thought to the use of manuals, a significant number viewed manuals as "a treatment protocol imposed by a third-party payer" (p. 336), or a technique that turns clinicians into technicians. Another study of therapists' satisfaction with a specific group treatment manual (Najavits et al., 2004) found that although the therapists viewed the treatment program positively and appreciated using a new approach, they reported that it took an average of 8 months to feel comfortable with the approach and they would not likely use the manualized approach, without modifications. The therapists felt that manuals did not offer sufficient guidance about treatment dilemmas and turned to supervision, rather than the manual, to address these issues.

Other writers challenge practitioners' critiques of manuals. Kendall and colleagues (1998) asserted that if a manual does not explicitly describe therapeutic techniques or relationships, clinicians must utilize their clinical skills. Further, they proposed that manuals should be used as guides to be applied with flexibility and creativity, and not as routinized procedures. According to this perspective, clinicians should be well versed with the treatment approach and the needs of the targeted population. Because manuals cannot address all potential treatment issues, supervision is vital for successful implementation. Finally, Galinsky and colleagues (2006) asserted that group leaders who use manuals must be skilled in group work, including the ability to foster relationships, nurture mutual aid, and pay attention to individuals' needs and group stages.

It is therefore prudent for researchers and practitioners to collaborate on the development of treatment manuals. Although treatment manuals are often developed by researchers, manuals need to be piloted in clinical settings and modified as needed. Continual modification is recommended as successful pilots are applied to more diverse populations (Galinsky et al., 2006).

THE DEVELOPMENT OF A MANUALIZED APPROACH TO GROUP WORK: CASE STUDY

In this article we describe the process of developing and piloting a group treatment manual for early adolescents with learning disabilities (LDs). Group treatment has been offered for many years at Integra, a children's mental health center in Toronto, Canada, that specializes in the mental health needs of children and youth with LDs. An approach to group work has been developed at the center (Mishna & Muskat, 2004) that utilizes self-psychology (Kohut, 1984), mutual aid (Gitterman & Shulman, 1994; Steinberg, 2004), and interpersonal group theory (Yalom & Lescz, 2005), and which accommodates the members' LDs (Mishna, 1996).

Group work is one modality offered at the center to address the struggles experienced by the children and adolescents receiving service. These include difficulties with academic performance, school failure, adjustment issues, depression, anxiety, social difficulties, and peer victimization (Cosden, 2001; Maag & Reid, 2006; Margalit & Al-Yagon, 2002; McNamara, Willoughby, Chalmers, & YLC-CURA, 2005; Morrison & Cosden, 1997; R. Pearl & Bay, 1999; Svetaz, Ireland, & Blum, 2000). Groups provide a setting for these children and youth to connect with others who also have LDs, to discuss their concerns, discover that others have similar struggles, and to address their psychosocial problems in a natural social environment (Mishna & Muskat, 2004).

The ability of individuals to understand and take control of their learning difficulties is a predictor of adult success (Raskin, Goldberg, Higgins, & Herman, 1999); this includes developing awareness of one's learning difficulties and strengths, and understanding the concept of "learning disability" and its specific academic implications. Best practice for students with disabilities includes delivery of programs that enhance self-determination (Wehmeyer, Field, Doren, Jones, & Mason, 2004). Self-determination includes self-advocacy, or awareness of one's rights to access support and accommodations, familiarity with needed accommodations, and the skills to communicate one's learning needs (Merchant & Gajar, 1997). The original group model developed at the center did not routinely or explicitly include discussion of the members' LDs or development of self-advocacy skills. It was important to incorporate discussion about LDs and self-advocacy in the revised group treatment model developed for the manual.

PILOT ONE: GROUP AS PART OF RESEARCH PROJECT

This manualized group approach was developed as one component of a school-based research project addressing the psychosocial needs of middle-school students with LDs. Together with university-based researchers and education personnel, the center was a partner in developing and implementing the project. The project objectives were to increase these students' understanding and ability to take control of their LDs; increase parents', teachers', and peers' understanding of LDs; and increase the support of the school environment in which the students function. The group model was developed to address the first objective, that is, increase the students' understanding and ability to take control of their LDs. The other two objectives are not discussed in this article.

Development of Group Manual

The manual was created primarily by an experienced agency-based group worker (BM) with the input and support of the university researcher. The manual was created using the "stage model" of manual development described by Carroll and Nuro (2002). Accordingly, development of a treatment manual is not considered a one-time event, but rather, a long-term process in which details of the approach are fine-tuned and enhanced based on pilot testing. The process includes a first stage during which an initial version of a manual is piloted, measures of adherence are created, and a training protocol is developed. In Stage 2, a series of controlled clinical trials are carried out and elements of the approach, either content or process related, are further developed. During Stage 3, the manual is piloted with diverse populations and is assessed for cost effectiveness. We are currently completing Stage 1 of development with respect to the "stage model."

The development of the manual was informed by (1) the group model used in the agency (Mishna & Muskat, 2004) and (2) the literature on best practices in working with students who have learning difficulties, including addressing self-awareness and self-advocacy (Raskin et al., 1999; Wehmeyer et al., 2004). Thus we included topics that had been used in the agency groups and were considered valuable and added topics that were identified in the literature, such as understanding LDs (Eisenman & Tascione, 2002;

C. Pearl, 2004), self-advocacy skills (Barga, 1996; Merchant & Gajar, 1997), and bullying experiences (Mishna, 2003, 2004). The manual was revised after use in the research project based on ongoing feedback from group leaders in the project and continues to be revised based on feedback from leaders of agency-based groups.

The primary focus of the manual is on the content of group sessions with the assumption that all the group leaders were trained in the group therapy model described previously (more details to follow). The group model described in the manual comprises 12 sessions (Muskat, 2004). The following information was presented for each session: check-in with members, outline of the session's purpose and objectives, didactic material /content, selected activities to illustrate the topic, snack, summary, wrap-up, and introduction of following week's theme. The first session included introductions including "ice breakers" and other activities to help the members become comfortable, brief review of the group purpose and goals, and development of group norms such as confidentiality and group safety as well as norms developed specifically by each group. The topics of the group sessions were as follows: (1) introductions, purpose, group rules, goal setting; (2) definition and description of LDs; (3) members' strengths and interests; (4) members' specific learning difficulties; (5) supports that help members learn and complete school work; (6) standing up for oneself/dealing with bullies; (7) role-playing and practicing standing up for oneself; (8) asking for help with school work; (9) learning to calm down and relax; (10) relaxation and problem-solving; (11) practicing lessons learned; and (12) summary, wrap-up, celebration, and awards. The aims of the sessions were to deliver content, utilize activities to illustrate content, allow for discussion, practice of self-advocacy skills, and promote fun. Information presented in the sessions, members' drawings and art, and worksheets used in sessions were placed in folders that were given to members at the end of the group. A list of relevant and accessible resources and readings were included at the end of each session.

Description of Group Intervention in the Research Project

The group comprised students in Grades 6–8, identified by special education staff of the school as having LDs, and invited by school staff to participate in the project. Participants were excluded if they scored in the clinical range for conduct problems on a standardized teacher report measure (Achenbach, 2001).

Each group was co-led by two leaders, one of whom was an agency social worker with clinical experience with this population and the other was a school-based social worker or psychologist. All of the leaders participated in a one-day training session on use of the manual as well as the group treatment approach used by the agency. The training was provided by one of the authors (BM) and comprised didactic and discussion modalities as well as analysis of videotapes of agency groups for children and youth with LDs. Throughout the project, a number of meetings were held with the group leaders, to obtain their comments and responses to the group process in general, and working with the manual more specifically.

Each group consisted of 12 weekly sessions, 60 minutes in length, with five to seven members. Groups were held in classrooms in the schools, either at lunchtime or during the school day.

Evaluation

The research group intervention was delivered to a total of 50 students in Grades 6 through 8, who participated in seven groups. All students were diagnosed with LD by a psychologist. The project as a whole was evaluated using quantitative and qualitative measures, to examine the students' self determination and adjustment. There were five waves of data collection (see Table 1).

The final sample of the whole project included 68 students (35 in immediate intervention and 33 in intervention withheld group). Of this sample, 18 withdrew from the study. Two students in the immediate intervention withdrew, as they no longer wished to participate; 16 students in the intervention withheld group withdrew (12 no longer wanted to participate and four moved). The final sample that received the intervention was 50 (33 in the immediate intervention, 17 in the intervention-withheld group).

We conducted individual interviews with selected participants in the group treatment to complement the quantitative data and tease out complex issues that other methods can overlook (Nastasi & Schensul, 2005). We used purposive sampling with respect to such variables as school and gender to obtain a range of experiences (Lincoln & Guba, 1985). Interviews focused on the participants' views of the group and the intervention. In addition, these students' teachers and parents were asked to participate in interviews to probe their impressions of the children's group involvement and of the overall program. Interviews were recorded and transcribed. We conducted interviews with 14 students, and their parents and teachers, for a total of 42 interviews. The student and teacher interviews took place at the schools and lasted approximately 1 hour, whereas the parent interviews were conducted over the phone. Several measures were taken to ensure

TABLE 1 Research Data Collection Schedule

Condition	Time 1	Time 2	Time 3	Time 4	Time 5
Immediate	Pretest	Posttest	6 mo. follow-up	12 mo. follow-up	18 mo. follow-up
Control/ Withheld	Pretest	Pretest	Pretest	Posttest	6 mo. follow-up

trustworthiness (Lincoln, 1995; Lincoln & Guba, 1985). The researchers' prolonged engagement through many years of practice and research with children who have LDs helped to build trust. Triangulation was achieved through the multiple perspectives obtained by interviewing the children as well as their parents and teachers. The data were analyzed through constant comparison to develop groupings of similar concepts of participants' perspectives (Creswell, 1998).

The findings of the individual interviews with the students who participated in the group, and their parents and teachers, suggest that the group contributes to ameliorating risk factors and promoting protective factors that are identified in the literature and that correspond with the aims of the group treatment. These factors include the students' knowledge of their LDs, increased ability to ask for help and self-advocate, and increased self-esteem and confidence. The details of the results are presented in manuscript separate article (Mishna & Muskat, this issue).

Participants' self-advocacy skills were assessed with The Self Advocacy Interview for Students, a 30-minute structured interview that evaluates knowledge of LDs, learning style, resources, accommodations, and communication skills (Brunello-Prudencio, 2001). Overall test–retest reliability was .875.

The means and standard deviations and F statistics for the Self Advocacy Interview (SAI) for the treatment and control groups are presented in Table 2.

The results indicate that (1) there were no significant differences in baseline SAI between the treatment and control groups, (2) both groups showed significant improvement in SAI from pretest/Time 1 to posttest/Time 2, and (3) there were no significant differences in posttest/Time 2 of assessment between the treatment and control groups.

We used general linear models repeated measure procedures to examine changes in self advocacy skills over five times of assessment. The results that are shown in Table 3 indicate that (1) at the one-year follow up, the treatment group made substantial gains in self advocacy knowledge and (2) students in the control-intervention group who received the self-advocacy

TABLE 2 Changes in Self-Advocacy Knowledge from Baseline to Posttest

Measure	Control ($N = 51$)			Withheld Intervention ($N = 35$)		
	M	SD	Range	M	SD	Range
SAI 1	29.0	6.11	11–42	28.33	5.38	18–39
SAI 2	32.8	6.22	12–46	33.15	5.11	23–43

Note. SAI 1 = Self Advocacy Interview Time 1; SAI 2 = Self Advocacy Interview Time 2.
Main Effect of Time: $F(1, 83) = 62.24$, $p = .000$, Eta$^2 = 0.43$; Time x Group Effect: $F(1, 83) = 0.72$, $p = .399$, Eta$^2 = 0.009$.

TABLE 3 Changes in Self-Advocacy Knowledge Across the Immediate and Delayed Intervention Groups

Measures	Immediate-Intervention (N = 33)			Withheld Intervention (N = 17)		
	M	SD	Range	M	SD	Range
SAI 1	29.17	6.077	18–39	28.20	7.51	11–42
SAI 2	32.98	6.224	23–43	30.47	6.81	12–46
SAI 3	30.28	7.637	23–44	29.20	7.66	13–42
SAI 4	35.14	5.187	20–41	34.73	5.24	20–41
SAI 5	35.00	4.914	25–44	35.00	4.91	26–42

Note. SAI 1 = Self Advocacy Interview Time 1; SAI 2 = Self Advocacy Interview Time 2; SAI 3 = Self Advocacy Interview Time 3; SAI 4 = Self Advocacy Interview Time 4; SAI 5 = Self Advocacy Interview Time 5.
Main Effect of Time: $F(1, 48) = 23.44$, $p = 000$, and $Eta^2 = .33$; Time x Group Effect: $F(1, 48) = 4.65$, $p = 004$, and $Eta^2 = .09$.

treatment after Time 3 of assessment also showed considerable increase in self-advocacy skills after the treatment.

These findings suggest that middle-school students with LDs can significantly increase their self-advocacy ability, an important protective factor. Results highlight the importance of adults discussing LDs with students, and understanding associated issues. As the project included the group, in addition to workshops for staff, teachers, and students, it is not possible to determine the isolated effects of the group component.

Pilot Two: Clinical Population

The process of piloting the manual led to adaptation and revisions, based on feedback from project group leaders collected throughout the project. Modifications include flexibility in the timing of delivery of content, development of activities linked to content, and less didactic material covered in each session. The revised manual was then piloted with the clinical population served by the agency.

With respect to timing of content and the nature of the material, leaders expressed frustration when they could not focus on a topic that a group member raised because the topic was assigned to another date in the manual. This critique corresponds to criticism in the literature about the tendency for manualized groups to be prescriptive rather than flexible according to the needs of the particular members. Accordingly, an explicit change to our manual entailed the room for leaders to adjust the timing of certain topics based on the needs of the group and issues raised by members. An example of this is the topic of bullying, which was assigned to be covered in the sixth session in the original manual. Leaders found this topic was often brought up in earlier sessions by members. The manual was then changed to encourage addressing this topic when it arose rather than holding it off to Session 6.

A second significant concern raised by group leaders was the large amount of didactic material and the limited number of activities offered in the manual through which the material could be communicated. The leaders found it difficult to engage the group members through this amount of material which they felt resembled school work. They also found that the children became restless in groups. This critique corresponds to the concern identified in the literature regarding lack of creativity, lack of attention to group dynamics, and inflexibility often found in manuals. Thus, effort was devoted to finding and developing appropriate activities that addressed the content in a way that engaged the group members and that fostered their active participation. For example, one group leader developed a bingo game about LDs. Another created a passport that used descriptions of specific learning difficulties to represent countries and had members receive stamps representing their specific struggles.

Four groups using the manual have been offered at the agency for its clinical population. The groups were co-led by agency staff members and university students. The agency staff members are experienced in individual, family, and group intervention, and the university students receive training in approaches used at the agency. The staff is accustomed to an unstructured, process-driven approach to group work, which typically consists of discussion and activities that foster socialization and communication (Mishna & Muskat, 2004). Therefore group leaders who did not participate in the school project were oriented to the new approach through participation in a day-long training session in use of the manual, provided by one of the authors (BM).

Historically, staff members have been quite pleased with the traditional approach to agency groups, in which group members are offered a positive social experience and the opportunity to experience mutual aid, which often results in members feeling better about themselves. Staff were not concerned about the fact that groups did not explicitly aim to increase members' understanding and coping with LDs. However, in agency-wide discussions on "best practice" with this population, this was identified as a gap in the group approach.

After using the manualized approach to group, the agency group leaders identified additional concerns with the approach. First, group members in agency groups are generally younger than the age group for which the manual was designed and are generally more active and distractible. Second, agency groups occur after school rather than during school hours, which is when they took place in the school-based project. Members attend agency groups after spending a day in school, and they have difficulty sitting still and absorbing information. The leaders also identified the 1-hour length of the agency groups as too short to effectively deliver the information presented in the manual.

Some leaders found it difficult to deliver the curriculum due to the concerns described above. Some did not want to make their own adaptation to the manual material and adhered quite rigidly to the material, albeit feeling dissatisfied. Others however, who were more supportive of the approach used in the manual, followed the core of the manual while altering activities to meet the developmental needs of their group members.

Some group leaders felt constrained by the structure of the manual and believed that children in groups needed and wanted to come to group to play and interact with others in an unstructured format. Some of these leaders resisted using the didactic material in their groups. However, other leaders appreciated the guidance provided by the manual. Several leaders approached the content quite creatively, for example, developing a "Guess the Learning Disability" game in which members asked questions of one another to discover what was written on pinned descriptions of LDs on their backs. Another leader had members create and videotape commercials in which the members practiced asking for help. Agency group leaders continue to use the manual in their groups and are involved in the process of making changes to the manual, eliminating and reordering some of the content, and creating a wider range of activities that address the content as well as the age and activity level of the group members.

Each agency group comprised six members for a total of 24 members. An evaluation is currently underway, utilizing qualitative and quantitative methods. The Self Advocacy Interview for Students, a 30-minute structured interview that evaluates knowledge of LDs, learning style, resources, accommodations, and communication skills (Brunello-Prudencio, 2001) that was used in the school-based project, is also being used in the agency pilot. Selected participants and parents will be interviewed as well to gain their views of the group experience. Following this, it is expected that there will be further decisions about the use of the manual and potential modifications to it.

PRACTICE PRINCIPLES IN DEVELOPING AND IMPLEMENTING A MANUAL

1. Work collaboratively with practitioners/group leaders: It is essential to obtain practitioners' views from the first conception of manual development, and to listen to and address their concerns. The ultimate objective is to assist practitioners to assume ownership of the group and the development and application of the manual. Even though the decision to utilize a manual may not be the choice of practitioners, it is imperative that their input and knowledge is recognized, appreciated, and taken into account. Practitioner input must be integral in the development of the approach, the crafting of the manual itself, and throughout the operation of the group.

2. Match the manual to the nature of the setting and to the characteristics of particular groups: The manual should take into account the specific culture of the setting, the theoretical approach used in the setting, and physical resources available for groups; for example, the room groups take place in, the time groups are offered, and the ability of members to sit still.

3. The manual should explicitly articulate and pay attention to group process as well as content: Although manuals are often associated with didactic content, it is imperative that manuals also contain information to assist in building, monitoring, and maintaining group process. The extent to which content or process is highlighted will be context dependent.

4. Stress that the leaders' creativity, skills, and knowledge of group work are vital: Encourage leaders to contribute their energy and creativity to enhance the group experience. Clarify that using a manual does not mean (1) throwing out group work knowledge, theories, and skills and (2) is not comparable to following a recipe. It is essential to communicate this throughout development and use of the manual to alleviate the group leaders' understandable resistance and fears.

5. Make it clear whether topics have to be followed sequentially: Although some manuals are constructed to build knowledge and skills from session to session, others contain material that can be covered in any order. Manuals should explain whether the order of presentation is essential and whether all content must be covered to achieve desired objectives.

CONCLUSION

In this article we report on the process of developing a manualized model of group treatment for early adolescents who have LDs, for students in a school-based intervention research project, and for clients in a community agency. Despite reluctance to adding didactic material and structured curriculum, group leaders in the research project and the agency were willing to pilot a new method of group work, which incorporated these components. Paradoxically, though many of the leaders stated that they did not enjoy leading the manualized group, they believed that most of the group members enjoyed and benefited from the experience.

The group leaders' feedback on the manual mirrored much of the criticism described in the literature. They were concerned about the suitability of the manual for a clinical population, the greater attention to content over group dynamics or mutual aid, and the manual's perceived restrictiveness. Similar to concerns expressed by Galinsky and colleagues (2006), group leaders believed incorrectly that inflexible adherence to the manual was essential, which in some cases resulted in the group leaders relinquishing some of their own group skills and creativity. Finally, the group leaders agreed that they would like to continue using the core of the manual, albeit with modifications.

The development of this manual will likely be a long-term process requiring much fine-tuning and enhancement. However, the end product represents a step toward employing the use of current best practice. This, we believe, is a step in enhancing the quality and effectiveness of group intervention.

ACKNOWLEDGMENT

This study was funded by a grant from the Social Sciences and Humanities Research Council of Canada. We acknowledge the support of the Toronto Catholic District School Board psychologists, social workers, teachers, and administrators, and the children and their parents, in particular Maria Kokai. We would like to thank Integra group leaders and administration, research assistants, and especially the research project coordinator Arija Birze.

REFERENCES

Achenbach, T. M. (2001). *Teacher Report Form*. Burlington, VT: University of Vermont, ASEBA .

Addis, M. E., & Krasnow, A. D. (2000). A national survey of practicing psychologists' attitudes toward psychotherapy manuals. *Journal of Consulting and Clinical Psychology, 68*(2), 331–339.

Association for the Advancement of Social Work with Groups. (2005). *Standards for social work practice with groups (2nd ed.). Re*-trieved February 22, 2007, from http://www.aaswg.org/Standards/standards%20single%20page%20layout1.pdf

Barlow, S. H., Burlingame, G. M., & Fuhriman, A. (2000). Therapeutic application of groups: From Pratt's "Thought Control Classes" to modern group psychotherapy. *Group Dynamics: Theory, Research & Practice, 4*(1), 115–134.

Barga, N. K. (1996). Students with learning disabilities in education: Managing a disability. *Journal of Learning Disabilities, 29*(4), 413–421.

Beutler, L. E. (2002). It isn't the size, but the fit. *Clinical Psychology: Science and Practice, 9*(4), 434–438.

Bratton, S. C., Ray, D., Rhine, T., & Jones, L. (2005). The efficacy of play therapy with children: A meta-analytic review of treatment outcomes. *Professional Psychology: Research and Practice, 36*(4), 376–390.

Brower, A. M., Arndt, R. G., & Ketterhagen, A. (2004). Very good solutions really do exist for group work research design problems. In C. D. Garvin, L. M. Gutiérrez, M. J. Galinsky (Eds.), *Handbook of social work with groups* (pp. 435–446). New York: Guilford Press.

Brunello-Prudencio, L. A. (2001). Knowledge and communication skills training for high school students with learning disabilities for the acquisition of self-advocacy skills. *Dissertation Abstracts International Section A: Humanities & Social Sciences, 62*(4-A).

Burlingame, G. M., Fuhriman, A., & Mosier, J. (2003). The differential effectiveness of group psychotherapy: A meta-analytic perspective. *Group Dynamics: Theory, Research and Practice, 7*(1), 3–12.

Burlingame, G. M., & Krogel, J. (2005). Relative efficacy of individual versus group psychotherapy. *International Journal of Group Psychotherapy 55*(4), 607–611.

Canadian Association of Social Workers. (2000). *CASW national scope of practice statement.* Retrieved July 22, 2005, from Ottawa: CASW Website: http://www.casw-acts.ca/Prac

Carroll, K. M., & Nuro, K. M. (2002). One size cannot fit all: A stage model for psychotherapy manual development. *Clinical Psychology: Science and Practice, 9*(4), 396–406.

Chorpita, B. F. (2002) Treatment manuals for the real world: Where do we build them? *Clinical Psychology: Science and Practice, 9*(4), 431–433.

Comer, E., Meier, A., & Galinsky, M. J. (2004). Development of innovative group work practice using the intervention research paradigm. *Social Work, 49*(2), 250–260.

Cosden, M. (2001). Risk and resilience for substance abuse among adolescents and adults with LD. *Journal of Learning Disabilities, 34*(4), 352–358.

Cramer-Azima, F. J. (2002). Group psychotherapy for children and adolescents. In M. Lewis (Ed.), *Child and adolescent psychiatry: A comprehensive textbook* (3rd ed., pp. 1032–1036). Philadelphia: Lippincott, Williams & Wilkins.

Cresswell, J. W. (1998). *Qualitative inquiry and research design: Choosing among five traditions.* Thousand Oaks, CA: Sage.

Eisenman, L. T., & Tascione, L. (2002). "How come nobody told me?" Fostering self realization through a high-school English curriculum. *Learning Disabilities Research & Practice, 17*(1), 35–46.

Galinsky, M. J., & Schopler, J. H. (1977). Warning: Groups may be dangerous. *Social Work, 22*(2), 89–94.

Galinsky, M. J., Terzian, M. A., & Fraser, M. W. (2006). The art of group work practice with manualized curricula. *Social Work with Groups, 29*(1), 11–26.

Gitterman, A., & Shulman, L. (1994). *Mutual aid groups, vulnerable populations and the life cycle.* New York: Columbia University Press.

Goodman, H., & Munoz, M. (2004). Developing social group work skills for contemporary agency practice. *Social Work with Groups, 27*(1), 17–33.

Hoag, M., & Burlingame, G. M. (1997). Evaluating the effectiveness of child and adolescent group treatment: A meta-analytic review. *Journal of Clinical Child Psychology, 26*(3), 234–246.

Kendall, P. C., Chu, B., Gifford, A., Hayes, C., & Nauta, M. (1998). Breathing life into a treatment manual: Flexibility and creativity with manual-based groups. *Cognitive and Behavioural Practice, 5*, 177–198.

Kohut, H. (1984). *How does analysis cure?* Chicago & London: University of Chicago Press.

Kulic, K. R., Horne, A. M., & Dagley, A. M. (2004). A comprehensive review of prevention groups for children and adolescents. *Group Dynamics: Theory, Research and Practice, 8*(2), 139–151.

Kurland, R., & Salmon, R. (2002). *Caught in the doorway between education and practice: Group work's battle for survival.* Plenary presentation at the 24th

Annual Symposium of the Association for the Advancement of Social Work with Groups, Brooklyn, NY.

Kurland, R., Salmon, R., Bitel, M., Goodman, H., Ludwig, K., Newman, E. W., et al. (2004). The survival of social group work: A call to action. *Social Work with Groups, 27*(1), 3–16.

Lincoln, Y. S. (1995). Emerging criteria for quality in qualitative and interpretive research. *Qualitative Inquiry, 1*(3), 275–289.

Lincoln, Y. S., & Guba, E. G. (1985). *Naturalistic inquiry.* Newbury Park, CA: Sage.

Maag, J. W., & Reid, R. (2006). Depression among students with learning disabilities: Assessing the risk. *Journal of Learning Disabilities, 39*(1), 3–10.

Mace, C. (2006). Setting the World on Wheels: Some clinical challenges of evidence-based practice. *Group Analysis, 39*(3), 304–320.

Macgowan, M. J. (2006). Evidence-based group work: A framework for advancing best practice. *Journal of Evidence-Based Social Work, 3*(1), 1–21.

Margalit, M., & Al-Yagon, M. (2002). The loneliness experience of children with learning disabilities. In B. Wong & M. Donahue (Eds.), *The social dimensions of learning disabilities: Essays in honor of Tanis Bryan* (pp. 53–75). Mahwah, NJ: Lawrence Erlbaum.

McDermott, F. (2003). Group work in the mental health field: Researching outcome. *Australian Social Work, 56*(4), 352–363.

McMurran, M., & Duggan, C. (2005). The manualization of a treatment programme for personality disorder. *Criminal Behaviour and Mental Health, 15*, 17–27.

McNamara, J. K., Willoughby, T., Chalmers, H., & YLC-CURA. (2005). Psychosocial status of adolescents with learning disabilities with and without comorbid attention deficit disorder. *Learning Disabilities Research & Practice, 20*(4), 234–244.

McNicoll, P., & Lindsay, J. (2002). Group work in social work education: The Canadian experience. *Canadian Social Work Review, 19*(1) 153–166.

Merchant, D. J., & Gajar, A. (1997). A review of the literature on self advocacy components in transition programs for students with learning disabilities. *Journal of Vocational Rehabilitation, 8*, 223–231.

Mishna, F. (1996). Finding their voice: Group therapy for adolescents with learning disabilities. *Learning Disabilities Research & Practice, 11*(4), 249–258.

Mishna, F. (2003). Learning disabilities and bullying: Double jeopardy. *Journal of Learning Disabilities, 36*(4), 336–347.

Mishna, F. (2004). A qualitative study of bullying from multiple perspectives. *Children & Schools, 26*(4), 234–247.

Mishna, F., & Muskat, B. (2004). I'm not the only one! Group therapy with older children and adolescents who have learning disabilities. *International Journal of Group Psychotherapy, 54*(4), 455–476.

Mishna, F., & Muskat, B. (2010). I'm not lazy; it's just that I learn differently: Development and implementation of a manualized school-based group for students with learning disabilities. *Social Work with Groups, 33*(02), 138–158.

Morrison, G., & Cosden, M. (1997). Risk, resilience and adjustment of individuals with learning disabilities. *Learning Disability Quarterly, 20*(1), 43–60.

Muskat, B. (2004). *Project Inside and Out: Enhancing self understanding in students with learning disabilities group work manual.* Unpublished manual, Integra, Toronto, Ontario.

Najavits, L. M., Ghinassi, F., Van Horn, A., Weiss, R. D., Siqueland, L., Frank, A., et al. (2004). Therapist satisfaction with four manual-based treatments on a national multi-site trial: An exploratory study. *Psychotherapy: Theory, Research, Practice, Training, 4*(4), 26–37.

Nastasi, B. K., & Schensul, S. L. (2005). Contributions of qualitative research to the validity of intervention research. *Journal of School Psychology, 43*(3), 177–195.

National Association of Social Workers. (1999). *Code of Ethics of the National Association of Social Workers approved by the 1996 NASW Delegate Assembly and revised by the 1999 NASW Delegate Assembly.* Retrieved April 30, 2008, from National Association of Social Workers Website: http://www.naswdc.org/pub/code/code.asp

Page, R. C., Weiss, J. F., & Lietaer, G. (2001). Humanistic group psychotherapy. In D. J. Cain & J. Seeman (Eds.), *Humanistic psychotherapies: Handbook of research and practice* (pp. 339–368). Washington, DC: American Psychological Association.

Pearl, C. (2004). Laying the foundation for self-advocacy: Fourth graders with learning disabilities invite their peers into the resource room. *Teaching Exceptional Children, 36*(3), 44–49.

Pearl, R., & Bay, M. (1999). Psychosocial correlates of learning disabilities. In V. L. Schwean & D. H. Saklofske (Eds.), *Handbook of psychosocial characteristics of exceptional children* (pp. 443–470). New York: Kluwer/Plenum.

Pollio, D. E. (2002). The evidence-based group worker. *Social Work with Groups, 25*(4), 57–70.

Pollio, D. E. (2006). The art of evidence-based practice. *Research on Social Work Practice, 16*(2), 224–232.

Raskind, M. H., Goldberg, R. J., Higgins, E. L., & Herman, K. L. (1999). Patterns of change and predictors of success in individuals with learning disabilities: Results from a twenty-year longitudinal study. *Learning Disabilities Research and Practice, 14*, 35–49.

Roback, H. B. (2000). Adverse outcomes in group psychotherapy. *Journal of Psychotherapy Practice Research, 9*, 113–122.

Scaturo, D. J. (2001). The evolution of psychotherapy and the concept of manualization: An integrative perspective. *Professional Psychology: Research and Practice, 32*(5), 522–530.

Shlonsky, A., & Gibbs, L. (2004). Will the real evidence-based practice stand up? Teaching the process of evidence-based practice to the helping professions. *Brief Treatment and Crisis Intervention, 4*(2), 137–153.

Steinberg, D. M. (2004). *The mutual-aid approach to working with groups: Helping people help one another.* New York: Haworth Press.

Svetaz, M. V., Ireland, M., & Blum, R. (2000). Adolescents with learning disabilities: Risk and protective factors associated with emotional well-being: Findings from the National Longitudinal Study of Adolescent Health. *Journal of Adolescent Health, 27*(5), 340–348

Ward, D. E. (2004). The evidence mounts: Group work is effective. *Journal for Specialists in Group Work, 29*(2), 155–157.

Wehmeyer, M. L., Field, S., Doren, B., Jones, B., & Mason, C. (2004). Self-determination and students' involvement in standards-based reform. *Exceptional Children, 70*(4), 413–425.

Weisz, J. R., Weiss, B., Han, S. S., Granger, D. A., & Morton, T. (1995). Effects of psychotherapy with children and adolescents revisited: A meta-analysis of treatment outcome studies. *Psychological Bulletin, 117,* 450–468.

Westen, D., Novotny, C. M., & Thompson-Brenner, H. (2004). The empirical status of empirically supported psychotherapies: Assumptions, findings, and reporting in controlled clinical trials. *Psychological Bulletin, 130*(4), 631–663.

Yalom, I. D., & Lescz, M. (2005). *The theory and practice of group psychotherapy* (5thed.). New York: Basic Books.

Teaching Evidence-Based Practice to Administrative Groups: The Professional Academy of Evidence-Based Practice

STEPHANIE KRAUSS

Shearwater Education Foundation,St. Louis, Missouri, USA

BARBARA LEVIN

George Warren Brown School of Social Work, St. Louis, Missouri, USA

As the field of social work moves toward the implementation of evidence-based practice, agencies require training, mentoring, and peer networking to ensure successful adoption. This article defines successful adoption as knowledge and competence in the process of evidence-based practice. Successful adoption is best accomplished through the education and training of organization teams comprising key leaders—executive staff and board members. The Professional Academy for Evidence-Based Practice described in this article is the training vehicle, designed through and as the task group work model.

THE DILEMMA

The field of social work is moving toward the formal implementation and adoption of evidence-based practice (EBP). Mullen and Streiner (2004) suggested that in the near future, government bodies, insurers, and accreditation bodies will require this methodology from their practitioners and/or funding recipients. As this trend toward a more scientific knowledge base continues, few agencies are receiving formal training on implementation strategies for practice. Although many agencies express a desire to learn EBP, few agencies have officially adopted its methodology (R. E. Drake et al., 2001). The purpose of this article is to describe a program proposed to meet this need for agency training.

The program is the collaborative effort between myself, a former educator, and a trained group worker. My colleague and I are a part of the George Warren Brown School of Social Work at Washington University in St. Louis, Missouri, which is known for its leadership in spearheading the educational training of EBP (Howard, McMillen, & Pollio, 2003). Through recent conversations, a shared apprehension pertaining to the adoption of EBP emerged. As such, this program, the Professional Academy of Evidence-Based Practice (hereinafter PAEP) is born out of this tension. All of our knowledge surrounding EBP seems to be University contained. Although the information and findings are promising, the articles are highly cerebral, and recommendations for practitioner training rarely include opportunities for practitioners to integrate their experiential and intuitive knowledge. The program seeks to combine the empirical gems retrieved from the existing literature on EBP, while placing high value and priority on the assets of the local practitioner.

PRACTITIONER RESPONSIBILITY TO ADOPT EVIDENCE-BASED PRACTICE

EBP is a social work methodology that enables social workers to use current best evidence to make professional decisions (Mullen, 2002). The effective use of this evidence is contingent upon the practitioner's ability to merge his or her experiential wisdom with empirical findings (Bricout, Pollio, Edmond, & McBride, 2008). Implementation is achieved when social workers are able to successfully practice their evidentially supported treatments and interventions (Gambrill, 2004).

The process of conducting EBP can be broken into five steps. By utilizing this process, the practitioner collects relevant evidence for practice and discovers any gaps in the literature. Just as individuals expect their doctors to correctly diagnose and treat an illness, based on most recent research, so social work practitioners should be expected to use available evidence when determining client care. The five-step process of EBP is as follows: (1) the practitioner identifies a social need, the practitioner forms that need into an empirical question; (2) the practitioner gathers all current and available literature relevant to this need; (3) the practitioner critically evaluates this literature; (4) merge findings into a practice situation; (5) the practitioner evaluates the success of the intervention (B. Drake, Hovmand, Jonson-Reid, & Zayas, 2007). When the community of social work practitioners engages in such a rigorous process, the credibility of the profession is promoted and the quality of services rendered is enhanced (Howard et al., 2003).

Within the field, there are some criticisms of EBP. A great apprehension of formal adoption is the creation of a "cookbook" method to solving social problems; practitioners fear that clients will be treated according to predetermined sets of measurement (Howard et al., 2003). The risk of such a rote and impersonal approach is eliminated by a practitioner's applied professional discretion to modify approaches to meet client needs.

Another criticism of this methodology is the financial and time constraint necessary to conduct EBP (Howard et al., 2003). This is a real barrier, because the collection, critique, and evaluation of evidence takes time, and access to databases can be financially burdensome. An individual practitioner must be willing to commit to these costs, because successful adoption of EBP within organizations is contingent on the establishment of certain support factors. These include, but are not limited to, the following: agency policies and procedures that promote the process of evidence-based research and ensure its fidelity, funding support from accreditation and supporting bodies, a structure for routine monitoring and assessment of gathered research, a receptivity toward developing dissemination materials (e.g., professional toolkits), finally, organizations must have practitioners or partners who have been trained in the EBP methodology (Mullen, 2002).

Social work practitioners have a unique responsibility in the promulgation of EBP. Their professional experience and wisdom enables them to critically evaluate evidence and identify otherwise hidden gaps in the literature. By reviewing the literature, some may choose to conduct the necessary research to substantiate specific social work practices. By using professional judgment, social work practitioners should be able to appraise EBPs for their utility, pragmatism, and validity (Howard et al., 2003). This can lead to the dissemination of useful and successful therapeutic approaches, which ultimately ensures more effective interactions between social worker and client.

PROGRAM DESIGN

The PAEP is a program designed by the Alliance for Building Capacity. The Alliance for Building Capacity is an initiative of the George Warren Brown School of Social Work at Washington University. The Alliance for Building Capacity is committed to the promotion of evidence-based training and practice, and out of this core value, PAEP was designed to meet an organization's need for education and training on the process of EBP. PAEP brings together those agencies that demonstrate a readiness to learn and successfully adopt EBP into their decision-making process. The PAEP program is constructed to bring local nonprofit agencies and Brown School faculty into professional dialogue and potential partnerships. The primary purpose of PAEP is to train the executive leadership of eligible community agencies in exemplar ways of conducting EBP; secondarily, PAEP is structured to create and sustain a network of the St. Louis agencies and academicians who practice this methodology. In the following sections, the proposed program design of PAEP is described in detail.

Group Work Orientation

PAEP is structured as a short-term task group. This evidentiary approach consists of the following three phases: (1) problem identification and assessment, (2) procedural planning for task implementation, and (3) termination (Reid & Fortune, 2003). In adherence to this three-phase model, PAEP will be divided into three 2-day seminars, occurring once per month; Seminar One is dedicated to the first phase and so on.

At PAEP, the executive leadership body, also known as the administrative team will represent their agency; these are the individuals who are responsible for agency advancements and improvements in service areas (Fatout & Rose, 1995). By bringing these administrative teams through the process of EBP, PAEP provides an opportunity for local agencies to improve their quality of care and to engage in current techniques of research and practice.

Goals and Expectations of PAEP

The Alliance for Building Capacity determined a set of program outcomes and expectations, to be achieved by each participating entity. First, PAEP is designed to function out of the Brown School and being as such, the following benefits have been identified for the Brown School community: (1) PAEP will serve as a way for the Brown School to engage in more organized and systematic relationships with the St. Louis community; (2) PAEP promotes the Brown School's mission to collaborate with agencies to improve their quality of services; (3) PAEP further promotes the Brown School mission by applying the results of the School's EBP research; (4) PAEP is designed to advance the successful implementation of EBP at the organizational level, something that the Brown School is committed to; (5) PAEP serves to catalyze partnerships between faculty members and local agencies; and (6) PAEP is a vehicle through which the Brown School can disseminate research findings on EBP.

Agency benefits are dependent upon each team's level of commitment. During the program, teams will be assigned specific tasks to bring them through the evidence-based process. By design, the completion and comprehensive understanding of the process will build a competence and confidence in the process of EBP. Unfortunately, some teams never coalesce, and their experience of tension or conflict leaves them unable to complete the entire process (McDermott, 2002). Predetermined goals for enrolled teams include the completion of several deliverables; these formal "take-aways" will provide a baseline for future research, or reference. Team assignments include the following: (1) the board chair and executive director's individual completion of the Alliance for Building Capacity Organizational Audit, to assess organizational capacity and cohesion; (2) A "Summary of Learnings" briefing prepared after Seminars 1 and 2, to be presented to a panel of Brown School faculty who are trained in the process of EBP; and (3) a prepared presentation of research findings for Seminar 3.

As an extension to the seminars, the Alliance for Building Capacity proposes biannual "Briefing Breakfasts" where PAEP graduates meet with program alumni, incoming participants, and involved Brown School faculty and staff. The Alliance for Building Capacity is committed to partnering enrolled agencies in long-term relationships with other agencies in their PAEP cohort, and the purpose of these meetings is to share findings, discuss problems, and support each other in the continued implementation of EBP. These breakfasts will be an informal venue for professional discourse on the challenges and successes of EBP adoption. Briefing Breakfasts will enrich the network of agencies in the St. Louis region that have been trained in the process, while additionally furthering the mission and values of the Brown School.

Who Should Attend?

In an effort to create a cohesive and strong community of trained practitioners, the Alliance for Building Capacity identified six criteria for participant eligibility. Each criterion for eligibility ensures agency commitment to the 3-month seminar and future implementation. The criteria for PAEP participation is as follows: (1) the administrative team demonstrates a readiness to share, assess, and evaluate their agency; (2) the agency holds 501(c)3 status; (3) the executive director and board chair (or board designee) both commit to attending all three seminars; (4) the agency has a Board of Directors who support the adoption of EBP; (5) participants have held their agency position for at least 6 months, preferably 1 year; (6) administrative teams are three persons at minimum and five persons at maximum; (7) all administrative teams include the executive director and designated board member. The Alliance for Building Capacity desires an agency's eagerness to implement, above a readiness to participate, and therefore ineligible agencies will be considered on an at-need basis.

Social context. PAEP cohorts will be homogenously grouped, according to the client population that they serve. According to Fatout and Rose (1995), task groups most benefit from partnering with agencies whose mission and values are compatible with their own. Being as such, PAEP programs will operate under the following five concentrations: health; mental health; gerontology; children, youth, and families; and social and economic development. These are the same concentrations that are offered through the Brown School curriculum; this is done to ensure the closest alignment between the research interests of participating Brown School faculty and the program participants. Additionally, as faculty members produce research within their concentrations, former participants will have easy access to these new empirical findings. Finally, the Alliance for Building Capacity believes that group dynamics are stronger and more unified when cohort teams experience a shared identity, a sense of collective mission, and interdependence with one another (Forsyth, 1999).

Structure of PAEP

In the program-planning phase, three structural issues have to be addressed. The first is whether administrative teams or the Alliance for Building Capacity determines the group process; the second is whether or not to define team roles; the tertiary issue is the delegation of group member responsibilities within the team and cohort.

For the PAEP program to be an evidence-based method of teaching the process of EBP, the program structure and curriculum must be replicable; as a result, constant monitoring, clear expectations, measurable outcomes, and periodic evaluations are imperative. Each team will have the flexibility to identify an agency-specific social need, but the seminar structures are designed by the Alliance for Building Capacity. Administrative team member roles will be determined by member positions within the agency. For example, the executive director of a participating agency will be accountable for ensuring task completion, and the designated board member will facilitate the simulated board presentation that occurs during Seminar 3. To address the third issue, the Alliance for Building Capacity has made targeted responsibilities for the executive director and designated board member. All other agency participants will be placed in support roles, with their tasks assigned by the executive director.

The facilitation of group time and any outside meetings will be the responsibility of the executive director; the official reporting of final decisions and group mediation will be the role of the designated board member. The combined efforts of all team members ensure that groups quickly accomplish tasks; the feedback provided by cohort teams and Brown School faculty and staff guarantees a satisfying experience (Rivas & Toseland, 1984).

Duration, Timing, & Frequency

PAEP is proposed as a time-limited program. The Alliance for Building Capacity is cognizant of agency time constraints; additionally, time-bound groups create novelty among teams, which can increase risk taking and experimentation (Fatout & Rose, 1995). Any device that increases appropriate risk taking and experimentation is a valuable asset to this program.

As aforementioned, PAEP is divided into three, 2-day seminars, occurring once per month. Seminar days will run during typical workday hours;

participants will be given a 1-hour lunch break, in addition to coffee and snack breaks throughout the day. The next section provides an overview of the organizational structure of each Seminar. The PAEP program is designed to run biannually, once during the fall academic semester and once during the spring academic semester; it is on a five-cycle rotation, with each semester dedicated to one concentration.

Seminar Descriptions

Initial evaluation. Prior to their arrival, each administrative team is responsible for completing the Alliance for Building Capacity's Organizational Audit. This tool assesses an organization in the following five focus areas: programs, management, governance, resources, and systems. Audit results will inform the Alliance for Building Capacity of each organization's level of maturation, in addition to its capacity within particular areas. The Alliance for Building Capacity will be able to draw from agency strengths to shape program facilitation; additionally, PAEP curriculum can be modified for certain administrative teams, or if necessary, entire cohorts.

Seminar 1: Introduction to evidence-based practice & problem identification. Seminar 1 is a time to shape teams and develop a cohort's culture (Fatout & Rose, 1995). During the first session, introductions will be made, team requirements addressed, and group goals discussed and established. Administrative teams will be encouraged to discuss their findings from the Organizational Audit; teams will also have an opportunity to discuss their excitement, hesitations, and questions about EBP. Throughout this time, the Alliance for Building Capacity will create effective ties between teams by summarizing the similarities that exist among participants; this is done to develop a trusting and open environment for continued sharing throughout all seminars (Fatout & Rose, 1995).

During the first part of this orientation process, administrative teams will be given an overview of EBP, including the historical, philosophical, and practice perspectives behind the methodology. By ensuring a general understanding of the methodology, participants will have a clearer idea of what to expect from the academy and how to use the process to meet agency needs. Additionally, administrative teams will participate in a variety of experiential exercises designed for group members to practice their assigned roles and responsibilities. This is a time for working relationships to develop and teams to begin coalescing around a common set of purposes and goals. As conflicts and questions arise, the executive director from each team is responsible for motivating his or her team to move forward, whereas the designated board member is responsible for working to resolve any issues at hand.

On the second day, the administrative teams decide on one social need to research by using the evidence-based process. As teams discuss their prospective social needs, they will be asked to identify any organizational supports that could help in the research process. The Alliance for Building Capacity will help by giving evidence-based verbiage around each team's chosen social need; each team will be responsible for devising an empirical question from their identified social need. Once this is formed, specific tasks will be assigned to each group member, to continue the evidence-based process. By the end of Seminar 1, teams have completed the first step of the evidence-based process through the identification of an agency-specific social need to research. Between Seminars 1 and 2, teams will complete the second step of the process, which is the gathering of all available and current evidence.

Prior to their arrival at Seminar 2, administrative teams must complete the tasks assigned to them during Seminar 1. If necessary, these tasks could have been revised, or even reassigned. In between these seminars, the Alliance for Building Capacity and involved faculty will behave as consultants for the teams. Additionally, each administrative team will be assigned one masters- or doctoral-level social work student to assist in their evidence gathering.

Seminar 2: Procedural planning for task implementation. Seminar 2 will be conducted as an exchange forum within teams and between teams. Groups will present their "Summary of Learnings" to a panel of evidence-based researchers and faculty. Throughout the first day, administrative teams will share their findings and receive feedback. As teams present their findings, panelists and administrative teams will be responsible for offering suggestions and assessments about the completed work. During this time, the Alliance for Building Capacity's role is to encourage the now self-governing teams to continue working toward their goals. At the end of this seminar, administrative teams will conduct a self-monitoring exercise; in this exercise, teams will create a list of concerns to address and questions to answer, before continuing on in the process (Fatout & Rose, 1995).

By the end of the 2 days, teams will begin critically evaluating their literature. To ensure quality implementation of the process, teams will receive support and ongoing counsel from a faculty researcher who is trained in EBP and who also shares similar interests. Between Seminar 2 and 3 each administrative team will be asked to set a date to begin Step 3 of the evidence-based process, which is the merging of their findings into practice. The Alliance for Building Capacity, student liaisons, and the involved faculty will routinely follow up with the teams and help to track their progress.

Seminar 3: Termination. The final Seminar will begin with team presentations of "Summary of Learnings" briefings to Brown School panelists. In this way, all teams will have an opportunity to receive feedback on the work conducted between Seminars 2 and 3. On the second day, the classroom will become a simulated boardroom where each team will give a formal presentation of their findings. Their presentations will include an overview of the chosen social need, a list of problem-solving strategies that were found in the evidence, methods for successful strategy implementation, ways that the client should profit from these new strategies, and the identification of any other needs that can be researched through the repeated process of EBP (Reid & Fortune, 2003). The first cohort's program officially will be terminated with a wine and cheese social. The social allows participants to celebrate their empirical achievements and informally network with the Brown School faculty, staff, students, and other program participants. In following semesters, program alumni will also be invited to attend this social. It is the hope of the Alliance for Building Capacity that agencies will network not only for professional development, but also to build a supportive community with one another and with the Brown School.

Evaluation

The Alliance for Building Capacity has designed the PAEP program with the goal of it becoming a replicable professional development program that meets the needs of local agencies that want to learn and build competencies in the process of EBP. To guarantee that this goal is met, constant and valid evaluation methods must be employed.

Participants will evaluate the training in a multitude of ways. Each participant will be given a midcourse and final self-evaluation, to evaluate program effectiveness, content utility, and overall satisfaction. Each team will be required to participate in a focus group, 3 or 4 months after the training. These focus groups will be conducted by the Alliance for Building Capacity. Groups will be asked about the utility of learned skills, components that could be improved, and program sessions that were most valuable. Additionally, agency application of EBP will be tracked by distributing short evaluations at each Briefing Breakfast.

Monitoring and evaluation will also be required of participating faculty. Panelists will be given self-evaluations following Seminars 2 and 3. Immediately following Seminars 2 and 3, focus groups will be held with student liaisons; students will be asked to evaluate training effectiveness and the success of each team's adoption with EBP. The Alliance for Building Capacity will use the information obtained to modify future trainings and facilitation.

Limitations

There are several limitations with the PAEP program proposal. The largest limitation is that program success is contingent on the preparedness, commitment, and enthusiasm of its participants. These three components must be critically assessed while the cohort culture is being formed and then monitored throughout the seminars. Program objectives and daily expectations must be clear and enforced. Another limitation is that the development of cohorts is dependent on the expressed need of agencies to receive training. Without successful marketing, PAEP may not attract a large enough pool of participants for each concentration, in which case, homogenous grouping would be impossible.

Additionally the possibility that an agency identifies a social need that has little to no available evidence also limits program success. If agencies encounter such gaps in the literature, they will be provided with two options. The first is that the agency chooses a new social need, with a plethora of published research material. The second option is that the agency gathers all evidence that is distally related to their specific need, and from this literature base teams can cull all pertinent evidence. With faculty consultation, they will be able to draw some relevant determinations for practice. Teams who encounter this particular limitation will be encouraged to explore opportunities for outside research to work toward closing this research gap.

The final limitation to the program design is the potential for poor facilitation. The composite nature of administrative groups demands that program facilitators be well versed in the evidence-based process and properly trained in group work facilitation. This includes the successful employment of facilitation interaction techniques, such as confronting, attending to, negotiating with, mediating between, summarizing for, and giving information to the whole group, administrative teams, and individual participants. The facilitator's ability to successfully carry out these techniques will determine the pace, tone, and culture of the program (Doel & Sawdon, 1999). Ultimately, his or her ability to lead the program can promote the success or failure of the entire program.

Implementation and Sustainability of PAEP

As with all program development, the implementation of PAEP is contingent on having a strategically focused implementation plan that includes resource development planning (human and capital), leadership commitment from the Brown School, a developed understanding of the competitive landscape, solid marketing, and communication strategies. Drawing on evidence-based management principles, PAEP can be launched within 8 months of securing sufficient resources and fiduciary support. Initial funding will be sought through grants, in particular from local foundations that have a designated focus on capacity building or EBP. A subgrant design would be most desirable, as it could be used to supplement agency costs for the time spent at PAEP. It would be provided to agencies on the agreement that they attend all three seminars, complete all tasks, and participate in follow-up evaluation and monitoring.

The Alliance for Building Capacity plans to leverage its community network and relationships to identify the first cohort and will aggressively seek out those organizations and school partners who offer the best chance for success. An outline of this outreach strategy may secure additional early-stage funding. Documenting and communicating outcome measures and benchmarks of success will influence next stage investments sought from foundations. Future strategies for revenue generation and program advancements are curriculum dissemination and the creation of a toolkit for facilitator training.

Today, PAEP is in its infancy. Conversations about the program have begun at the University and community levels. The formal launching of PAEP is contingent on the approval of University stakeholders, but program success is contingent on the buy-in and commitment of community practitioners.

CONCLUSION

Successful implementation of EBP and improved client outcomes is dependent on a well-trained professional staff, in specific interventions and the process of EBP. The Professional Academy of Evidence-Based Practice is the first of its kind to address this training need in a format that reflects and respects the evidence of successful group work practice. The evaluation of training outcomes will inform our work, further the field, and inspire new research, which will lead to an increased evidence base.

REFERENCES

Bricout, J. C., Pollio, D. E., Edmond, T., & McBride, A. M. (2008). Macro practice teaching and curriculum development from an evidence-based perspective. *Journal of Evidence-Based Social Work, 5*, 597–621.

Doel, M., & Sawdon, C. (1999). *The essential groupworker*. Philadelphia: Jessica Kingsley Publishers Ltd.

Drake, B., Hovmand, P., Jonson-Reid, M., & Zayas, L. H. (2007). Adopting and teaching evidence based practice in masters level social work programs. *Journal of Social Work Education, 43*(3), 431–446.

Drake, R. E., Goldman, H., Leff, H. S., Lehman, A. F., Dixon, L., Mueser, K. T., et al. (2001). Implementing evidence-based practices in routine mental health service settings. *Psychiatric Services, 20*(4), 6–8.

Fatout, M., & Rose, S. R. (1995). *Task groups in the social services*. Thousand Oaks, CA: Sage.

Forsyth, D. R. (1999). *Radical casework: A theory for practice*. Sydney, Australia: Allen & Unwin.

Gambrill, E. (2004). Contributions of critical thinking and evidence-based practice to the fulfillment of ethical obligations of professions. In H. E. Briggs &

T. L. Rzepnicki (Eds.), *Using evidence in social work practice: Behavioral perspectives* (pp. 3–19). Chicago: Lyceum.

Howard, M. O., McMillen, C. J., & Pollio, D. E. (2003). Teaching evidence-based practice: Toward a new paradigm for social work education. *Research and Social Work Practice, 13*(2), 234–259.

McDermott, F. (2002). *Inside group work.* Crows Nest, Australia: Allen & Unwin.

Mullen, E. J. (2002). *Evidence-based knowledge: Designs for enhancing practitioner use of research findings.* Paper presented at the fourth International Conference on Evaluation for Practice, University of Tampere, Tampere, Finland.

Mullen, E. J., & Streiner, D. L. (2004). The evidence for and against evidence based practice. *Brief Treatment and Crisis Intervention, 4*(2), 111–121.

Reid, W. J., & Fortune, A. E. (2003). Task-centered practice: An exemplar of evidence-based practice. In A. R. Roberts & K. R. Yeager (Eds.), *Foundations of evidence-based social work practice* (pp. New York: Oxford University Press.

Rivas, R. F., & Toseland, R. W. (1984). *An introduction to group work practice.* New York: Macmillan.

Motivating Clients in Treatment Groups

SHELDON D. ROSE

University of Wisconsin-Madison, Madison, Wisconsin, USA

HEE-SUK CHANG

SungKongHoe University, Seoul, Korea

The purpose of this article is to describe a set of clinical principles for enhancing the motivation of participants in treatment groups. These principles are derived from the motivational-related research on therapy, the authors' own clinical experiences, and anecdotal evidence. The suggested strategies are aimed at improving the quality of treatment goals, enhancing clients' participation in therapy, acceptance of their problems, and working on resolving them. The underlying assumption is that ambivalence about therapy is normal and must be dealt with before treatment goals can be achieved.

INTRODUCTION

When most clients enter a treatment group for the first time they are often anxious, afraid of what others might think of them, and hesitant to expose their flaws to therapists or to other group members. For the most part, the entering clients can be regarded as ambivalent about the nature of the experience and the demands that they expect will be made on them. Above all, they are often poorly motivated to work on the very problems that brought them to the group. This lack of motivation is particularly apparent in groups of involuntary clients, such as delinquents, men who batter, prisoners, and those who abuse alcohol and drugs. However, even in voluntary groups, this ambivalence is often detectable. The types of behavior often observable in clients at early sessions are reluctance to speak, anger about being in treatment, denial of the problems, setting themselves apart from the others in the group, speaking only to the therapist, failure to disclose anything about themselves, and a reluctance to develop goals, treatment plans, or homework tasks.

The popular definition of *motivation* is the readiness of the client to participate actively in the treatment process and work toward formulating and achieving goals. Miller and Rollnick (1991) defined *motivation* as "the probability that a client will enter into, continue and adhere to a change strategy" (p. 19). That is, the commitment to change can be used interchangeably with motivation, and resistance is viewed as motivation's antithesis.

There are roughly two different kinds of approaches to viewing a client's motivation. The first approach considers motivation to be an internal disposition of the individual. From this individualistic standpoint, motivation is explained by one's personality traits or psychological qualities. The other perspective sees that motivation is rather an interpersonal process and considers social factors and personality characteristics. The latter approach has more direct implications for group counseling. The degree of motivation may find its causes not only in the learning history and attitudes of the client, but also in the client's pattern of interaction with the group therapist and other clients in the group. Motivation is not purely an internal psychological phenomenon but may rather be a function of the group and other contemporary social events.

Not all groups require a focus on motivation. In the experience of many practitioners, strategies for building the cohesion of groups are often sufficient to motivate the clients to participate, to set meaningful goals, and to try out new modes of behaving. In other cases, failure to focus seriously on the lack of motivation results in failure of treatment.

The role of motivation in behavior change is obviously crucial. Burke, Arkowitz, and Dunn (2002), in their review of 26 outcome studies, found the noticeable impact of motivational treatment on target behavior change. Inadequate motivation is also a major reason for dropping out of treatment (e.g., Stewart & Montplaisir, 1999). Zweben and Zuckoff (2002) reported mounting evidence of a relationship between treatment retention and better outcomes. In comparing recidivism rates of treatment completers versus noncompleters, batterers who left during treatment had higher rates of repeat violence, from one third to two thirds (Dutton, 1986; Edleson & Grusznski, 1989).

The purpose of this article is to present some clinical principles for enhancing the motivation of clients in the group and the ways in which some of these principles are implemented in the group to increase motivation. The skills outlined below are compatible with a cognitive-behavioral approach as well as with other, goal-oriented group techniques (see, e.g., Rose, 1998). It should be noted that most of these principles can be implemented during the course of therapy regardless of the group type as later examples will demonstrate.

PRINCIPLES OF ENHANCING MOTIVATION

Based on anecdotal reports and motivation research concerning individual treatment, practice theorists have developed a number of recommendations for group therapists to increase motivation among clients in the group. In addition, the unique aspects of the group lend itself to motivational enhancement. Insufficient attention to the norms of the group may also present some threats to motivation. It is worth noting that in the applications of these strategies, one must not ignore other activities that constitute the overt focus of the group. These include assessment, goal setting, group interventions, and planning for generalization.

The level of motivation in many instances overlaps with but is not the same as group cohesion. *Group cohesion* has been loosely defined as the mutual attraction of the clients to each other, to the goals of the group, and to the leader. This tripartite definition would be useful to the development of strategies for enhancing motivation. A group that can fulfill the needs or expectations of individuals is rewarding and leads to clients' attraction to the group, which in turn increases the level of motivation of the clients. If cohesion involves an increase in interpersonal rapport, it is likely that the clients will evolve and comply with change strategies provided by the group therapist. Also, success in change strategies will further increase the cohesion or the attraction of the group for its clients. Thus, the principle of enhancing motivation is usually closely connected with increasing the cohesion of the group. On the other hand, in those groups in which the cohesion is high, but preliminary individual goals are aimed at increasing the pleasure of group activities rather than on working toward change goals, the high cohesion may be an impediment to motivation to working toward positive change.

This article identifies two sets of principles. The principles in the first set represent effective clinical group treatment practice and indirectly enhance motivation. A total of 10 strategies suggested for group therapists are the following: (1) creating structures that promote broad and relevant participation, (2) eliciting and clarifying goals, (3) modifying other group structures or processes that interfere with prosocial change, (4) maximizing opportunities for personal choices, (5) practicing empathy, (6) giving clear information, (7) demonstrating an active helping attitude, (8) giving and receiving constructive feedback, (9) creating a reinforcing milieu in the group, and

(10) reducing interpersonal threats and arguments with individuals and the group.

The second set of principles more specifically directed toward enhancing motivation include (1) normalizing resistance and ambivalence, (2) weighing the costs and benefits of present behavior, (3) eliciting and reinforcing self-motivational statements, (4) removing barriers to active client involvement in treatment, (5) ongoing measurement of the level of motivation, and (6) follow-up contacts.

Let us discuss each of the clinical principles in terms of their impact on motivation not only as they are applied by the group therapist, but also as they are presented to clients in the group.

Principles that Indirectly Enhance Motivation

Creating structures that promote broad and relevant participation. Without participation, clients do not feel they belong to the group. If some participate and others do not, resentment often arises among clients. Self-disclosure can occur only through group participation. Only through participation can one receive the approval of one's peers. Yet, many clients, perhaps because of fear of disapproval, initially have a wait-and-see attitude, which, if not dealt with, results in long silences or irrelevant chattering.

Clients in the group who are unable to participate in the group activities and who impede group locomotion toward the completion of the task are much less attracted to the group and feel a stronger desire to terminate membership (Yalom, 1985). For example, Sethna and Harrington (1971) revealed that the most common cause of lapsing is the anxiety associated with participation in group therapy.

The therapist can use a number of strategies in the first group session to encourage broad and relevant participation. In particular, one exercise is used in which clients interview each other in pairs about family backgrounds, work experiences, personal interests and other recreational activities, previous treatment experiences, and their reasons for being in the group. Because the therapist is not present in these pairs, even the most reluctant clients feel comfortable talking. Then, each client, using notes collected in the paired interviews, introduces her or his partner to the rest of the group. In this way, very early in treatment, all clients have participated to roughly same extent, taken the first step at a safe and low level of self-disclosure, talked about themselves, and talked about someone else. There has been no opportunity for critical feedback. Even poorly motivated clients are able to follow these simple instructions and become involved.

During the rest of treatment, the group therapist makes use of other subgroup exercises to increase the participation of all the clients around increasingly demanding and self-revealing topics. Although such participation does not assure an increase in motivation, it is a prerequisite condition.

Eliciting and clarifying goals. The lack of direction in most non-goal-oriented groups is often responded to by passivity and disinterest, especially by the inexperienced group client. Therapy without goals creates a lack of structure, which is further anxiety producing. The explicitness of the method for goal attainment affects an individual's liking the group (Yalom, 1985) as well as his or her continuance–discontinuance status (Bernard & Drob, 1989). Bednar, Melnick, and Kaul (1974) argued that unclear goals and ambiguous group structure in the initial stage of the group retard early group development and contribute to premature client dropouts.

It is often premature to set specific goals in the first several sessions, before the clients know what the group has to offer and before they have explored what might be important for them. However, it is desirable for the therapist to make explicit the shared goal of establishing concrete individualized goals. This is an effective way of orienting the group to its central activity.

In goal-oriented groups, initial general goals are for the most part determined by the theme of the group, such as reducing alcohol abuse, eliminating violence toward partners, or improving relationships to significant others. Specific or situational goals are usually determined by each client with the help of the group and the group therapist. They may make suggestions to each other, providing a number of alternatives, and they may help evaluate consequences, but the final decision must be that of each client. The group therapist trains the clients in appropriate formulation of goals by means of a group exercise and multiple examples. The group therapist develops with the group a menu of goals that clients might work on. Then each of the goals is edited to fit the criteria for effective goal formulation.

All clients are instructed to select their own goals, either from the menu developed by the group or from their own experiences. After that, each person, one by one, gets feedback from the other clients in the group as to the appropriateness of these goals in terms of her or his larger purpose of being in the group and of the correctness of the formulation. Each client must be able to state that her or his goals are realistic and important before being encouraged to work toward achieving them. Although the other clients may encourage alternate goals, the ultimate choice, protected by the group therapist, is that of the given target client.

A moderate level of motivation may be necessary before relevant goals can be set. But as clients work on goal setting, motivation to work toward these goals appears to be further enhanced, provided that the small steps toward the goals are observable. In fact, group goal-setting studies (O'Leary-Kelly, Martocchio, & Frink, 1994) demonstrate the positive effect on group performance of assigned goals, which are motivational. The long-range, vaguely formulated goal may be too far in the future or too elusive to demonstrate steady progress, and as a result it may be a source of frustration that detracts from motivation. According to Wright and Kacmar (1994), goal specificity is the only main effect that lowers performance variance. For this reason, at least initially in groups, the goal-setting focus is on short-term, highly specific goals that are clearly linked to larger long-term goals. For example, in a group of alcohol abusers, several clients selected the goal of finding and participating in at least one nondrinking recreational activity on a regular basis.

Modifying other group structures or processes that interfere with prosocial change. Group structures or processes either interfere with or enhance individual or shared motivation. For example, a group of men who batter may have the shared belief that a real man, no matter how trivial the external annoyance, never lets anyone push him around. Failure to identify these shared values and to facilitate a critical analysis of them may result in little change, regardless of the intervention strategies employed. As part of critical analysis of stressful situations, cognitive restructuring techniques may be used (see Rose, 1998, Chapter 10 for a discussion how these are used in groups).

As group problems arise, helping the group to deal with those problems without blaming any one individual reduces the threat implied in group interaction, increases cohesion, and enhances the motivation of the clients, because they can observe problems of common concern being solved. Clients note that it is possible to deal with situations that make one uncomfortable without going on the attack. More specifically, therapists can resolve a group problem by (1) identifying the problem; (2) finding a shared description of that problem; (3) having each person, including the group therapist, look at his or her contribution to the problem; (4) generating alternative strategies for dealing with the problem; and (5) evaluating, selecting, and carrying out a solution (for examples, see Rose, 1998).

Common group problems include uneven distribution of participation, domination by one or two persons of the agenda of the session, excessive and inappropriate negative feedback, interpersonal conflict, fixed subgroup formation, and low cohesion. All of these group problems depress the motivation of the participants and are dealt with as they occur.

Maximizing opportunities for personal choices. If decisions, interpretations, goals, and advice are thrust upon the client, he or she is less committed than if the client feels free to choose by himself or herself. As seen above, clients ideally choose their own goals from a list generated by themselves often with the help of the group participants. Wherever possible, any recommendation, advice, or suggestion for action or change is offered in the form of options to be chosen by the client with a given problem.

The group therapist encourages the group to offer each client a number of different possibilities (a menu), which she or he must evaluate and then choose from. Just as with goals, advice is usually developed by means of brainstorming. In this group technique, once the problem is formulated, everyone writes down one or more ideas for dealing with the problem or achieving the goal. These are read one at a time to the client with the problem without any evaluation. Then, each potential goal or piece of advice is evaluated. The ultimate choice of action belongs solely to the target client. The group therapist and clients serve as consultants. The client is offered a number of possible formulations of the problems, goals, techniques, and plans for generalizing change much in this manner. In this way, clients not only make choices—they make informed choices.

Practicing empathy. *Empathy* has been defined in many different ways (Duan & Hill, 1996). For the purposes of this article, *empathy* refers to the communication to another of what the other person is experiencing, in a given situation, while showing understanding and acceptance. It is usually communicated through reflective statements. High levels of empathic functioning by individual therapists appear to be associated with low levels of resistance (Miller & Rollnick, 1991). It is highly likely that the same is true in group therapy. A positive therapeutic relationship plays a significant role in the development of cohesion. Although empathy is not directly measured, Antonuccio, Lewinsohn, and Breckenridge (1987) discovered that therapists who are rated as warmer are more effective at generating cohesive group interaction. Beckham (1992) revealed that dropouts evaluated their therapists as less warm, empathic, and genuine than nondropouts did. Murphy and Cannon's study (1986) also demonstrates that the formation of a good therapist–client relationship early in group therapy reduced the dropout rate. High levels of therapist warmth or caring may create a trusting, safe atmosphere that tends to enhance motivation and maintain clients in the group. Whenever clients reveal deeply experienced feelings in difficult situations, the therapist reflects the feelings she or he is perceiving and indicates that she or he finds them understandable. Statements such as, "It sounds like you__," "You're feeling __," "It seems to you that __," are used. The therapist also indicates an understanding of the behaviors that seem to be correlated with the feelings. This attitude of understanding does not mean the therapist or other clients in the group cannot differ from a given client. However, an empathic statement of understanding must precede an expression of differences either by the therapist or by the other clients in the group.

In groups, empathic responses by the clients to each other must also occur if a similar result is to be obtained. Because this is not a generally practiced skill, it may be necessary for the therapist to teach it to the clients, especially in groups in which clients are given to premature advice or problem solving.

An exercise can be used in which one client interviews another, while a third person serves as an observer. The topic is a recent stressful event or frustrating day. The interviewer is instructed to use reflective statements and other expressions of empathy, to avoid advice, and to show understanding. The roles shift twice, and then the subgroup discusses what the interviewers did well, and how they felt in the process.

Another way to teach the clients is for the group therapist to provide them with a series of vignettes that reflect situations encountered by people similar to the clients. The therapist after demonstrating effective ways to respond in the first examples, asks clients to reflect on the feelings of the individual in each of the remaining situations, and to share their impressions with each other. Then the group therapist encourages the clients to describe their own feelings in specific, recent stressful or anger-inducing situations. After each person explains the situation, the group therapist has the other clients write down what the target person has just said, as well as the feelings communicated when that person said it. The clients read their versions to the target person, who indicates which of the statements he thinks best reflects the meaning and the associated feelings of his statement.

Giving clear advice. Miller and Rollnick (1991) recommended that as clear advice is given and received by the client, motivation is enhanced. However, the advice should be requested by a client. In our experience, unsolicited advice or unclear advice has a lowering effect on motivation.

The therapist must make sure the clients in the group have learned how to give advice in the form of possible statements of what one could, rather than should, say or do under the conditions that the target person has described. The therapist first models how the advice should be given.

The group therapist does not elicit advice until the problem is clear. The therapist asks the other clients in the group whether the problem as stated by the client is clear to them, and what more they might need to hear from the client to understand it. The other clients are then asked to write down what advice they would give to the target client, and then each client gives written advice to the target client, adhering to the criteria for good feedback. It is only then that advice is given.

Demonstrating an active helping attitude. As we review the above and the following principles, it is clear that the group therapist plays an active helping role in the treatment process. We found that clients in groups are sometimes severely upset by the absence of help from the therapist, and by the therapist's failure to protect clients from confrontations by other clients in the group. More than other factors, a therapist's favorable attitude toward the client is crucial to predicting continuance in group treatment (Bostwick, 1987).

The group therapist demonstrates by attitude an active interest in all the clients' welfare. This attitude serves as a model for the clients in the group in helping each other. If a person asks for a specific kind of help, the group therapist assists in regard to the problem or refers the client to an alternative resource. Similarly, the clients in the group have information that might be helpful to the target client. This active helping attitude is in contrast to the attitude of the passive group leader who merely comments from time to time and leaves the group solely to its own devices.

Specifically, the therapist actively helps the clients in the group set goals, creates opportunities for them to make choices, helps them to develop advice for themselves and each other, gives them training in new behaviors, and creates conditions that optimize the possibility of enhancement of their motivation.

Giving and receiving constructive feedback. One of the advantages of group therapy is the rich source of feedback available to each client from other clients in the group. Feedback is intimately related to motivation. If misused, feedback can drive the client out of the group or create unbearable anxiety of the recipient, thus lowering motivation. If used constructively, feedback helps clients experience personal growth, satisfaction, and a sense of learning about themselves, which in turn enhances motivation. Feedback is usually used after a discussion or analysis of a stressful situation experienced by one of the clients, after role-play in which the client tries out a new way of dealing with a situation, and as part of the evaluation of the effectiveness of a given client's goal or plan for change.

One way of reducing the negative effects of feedback and enhancing its motivating aspects is for the therapist to teach clients directly how to give and receive constructive feedback. Exercises are used in which clients practice giving feedback first to the group therapist and then to each other, while adhering to the following set of prescribed criteria:

1. Give positive feedback first, then critical feedback.
2. Be specific in your comments (comment on behavior, not traits).
3. Critical feedback should be in the form of suggested alternatives to be considered.
4. Use "I" statements or give feedback as personal opinion.
5. Don't speak for group or higher authority.
6. Avoid absolute statements such as "never" or "always."
7. State criticism as hypothesis.
8. Avoid sarcasm/irony.
9. Avoid moral evaluative judgments.
10. Cite observable evidence or provide examples when possible.
11. Give clients permission to ignore suggestions, revise them or incorporate them as they choose.

Whenever feedback occurs in ongoing interaction, the therapist reinforces constructive and appropriate feedback and asks clients to rephrase inappropriate feedback. Similarly, exercises are used to train clients to receive all kinds of feedback to reduce the effect of negatively formulated critical feedback.

Creating a reinforcing milieu. Another form of communication is mutual reinforcement that serves as a motivation-enhancing technique. R. Liberman (1970) used two matched outpatient therapy groups to demonstrate that the systematic use of social reinforcement can increase group cohesiveness. The experimental therapist was trained to prompt and reinforce clients' statements that reflect cohesiveness. Comments made in the group that expressed approval of other clients were noted by the therapist. With expressions of praise, the therapist supported the clients' cohesive statements and encouraged them to make additional observations when appropriate. The results indicated that participants in experimental groups showed significantly more cohesiveness and were more group centered than participants in the comparison group. In spite of the significant role of the therapist, the study also found that the therapist was not the sole determiner of group interaction because, as time went on, the clients in the group themselves prompted and reinforced each other's behaviors. Budney, Higgins, Radonovich, and Novy (2000), in randomized clinical trials, demonstrated that adding a voucher-based incentive program to behavioral intervention reduced marijuana use among clients to a greater degree than those receiving either motivational or cognitive-behavioral therapy alone.

Reducing interpersonal threats to and arguments with individuals and the group. The group is a threatening and anxiety-producing environment for most participants. Threats create anxiety, which reduces the cohesion of the group and the motivation of the clients. It is necessary as early as possible to reduce the threat most clients experience in the face of potential criticism and negative peer feedback. This interpersonal threat is dealt with in the above-mentioned exercises and through therapist modeling. Many clients regardless of the presenting problem have poor social skills, and a few have social phobias. In addition to feedback training, to decrease the anxiety that the experience of being in a new group engenders, only gradual self-disclosure is encouraged. If clients reveal too much about themselves and their concerns too early, they often feel guilty and subject to unexpressed criticism, while the others are frightened by the excess of any one client too early in treatment. Because confrontation by others often has the same effect as punishment on a given client, premature confrontation is replaced by reflective statements. Clients are also discouraged from confronting each other in early sessions. M. A. Lieberman, Yalom, and Miles (1973) found that one of the principal reasons people dropped out of groups is that they feared attack or confrontation by the group, which suggested that confrontative techniques should be restricted until later in the group's development. Self-confrontation is another matter. The therapist may ask what meaning a given client gives to his or her own behavior. Likewise, the labeling of a client behavior by the other clients, which may be experienced as confrontation by the targeted client, is avoided. The use of diagnostic categories or any global descriptions of the negative characteristics of the clients is discouraged. Keeping the interaction essentially explorative, descriptive, specific, positive, and reflective, rather than confrontative and labeling, enhances the cohesion and the motivation of the group (Duan & Hill, 1996).

If a client does not accept a given goal or piece of advice, some group therapists argue with the client or encourage others in the group to argue with the given client, because peer group pressure is often an effective device for gaining the agreement of a client. Such argumentation goes against the principle of choice. Moreover, such pressure from the group may serve as either a threat or an aversive stimulus that would serve to decrease motivation. As a result, it is recommended that the group therapist not permit the clients to argue with the target person as a means of convincing the given person of the wrongness or rightness of his or her opinion or action. It is sufficient to hypothesize a different explanation or justification or strategy than that of the target client, or to encourage the group to do so. However, the more the other group members argue with a given client, the more defensive that client usually becomes. The group therapist will often recommend alternative ways of reasoning or performing and provide evidence for the clients' respective positions as alternatives. However, the group therapist ideally always reminds the target client of his or her choice and protects that choice from any group pressure.

Principles That Directly Enhance Motivation

The above principles represent good group work practice that indirectly has a bearing on motivation. The following principles suggest concrete strategies that deal directly with the enhancement of motivation.

Normalizing ambivalence and resistance. As noted earlier, almost all clients in treatment groups experience ambivalence and some degree of resistance to participating in the treatment. As early as the first session, it is necessary for the therapist to discuss the common nature of ambivalence toward change or receiving help. Some clients in the group may have perceived that they have had bad experiences with helping professionals. The clients are encouraged to talk about such experiences without passing judgment on the other professionals. They are asked to read a case example of a client who explicitly expresses ambivalence about coming to treatment. The clients are asked to discuss in small subgroups how they are different than and similar to the client in the example, in terms of their feelings about the group and what they are thinking. The clients in the group are asked to provide examples of ambivalence to change or treatment in previous settings. Based on the discussions of the case and previous experiences, the clients in the group usually conclude that ambivalence seems to be a common experience as one enters treatment one knows little about. The group therapist also notes that even as the group progresses, this ambivalence may not completely disappear. In general it seems to come and go depending on events in their lives and in the group, but it will usually reduce in intensity as clients have successful experiences in the group.

| Advantages of maintaining behavior | Disadvantages of maintaining behavior |
| Disadvantages of changing behavior | Advantages of changing behavior |

A

FIGURE 1 A Balance Scale.

Weighing the costs and benefits of present behavior. To provide a picture of the dynamic nature of their ambivalence, the clients are assisted in developing a balance scale (see Figure 1). The first step is to brainstorm with the clients the advantages of their present behaviors. While brainstorming, no discussion of alternatives or disadvantages is permitted. In this way, the clients in the group can see that the therapist and fellow clients in the group understand the importance or centrality of the behavior in their lives. Moreover, the clients are usually accustomed to people immediately telling them to stop doing what they are doing. The group therapist summarizes the list of advantages developed by the clients. The next step is for the group therapist to encourage the clients to look at the consequences of each other's present behaviors as they impinge on their general life goals. One exercise that is helpful is to have each client consider all the things he or she wants to do or achieve in the next 10 years. The group then discusses in what way the client's present behavior interferes with the achievement of any or all of these life goals.

Another exercise requests that each person present one argument for getting rid of the undesirable behavior, whether the given client is prepared to do so at that time or not. Each client, one at a time, adds an additional argument for change to those of the target person, until all arguments have been presented. The target client summarizes the arguments that are most convincing. During this discussion, the group therapist is careful to elicit opinions as to disadvantages, consequences, and the need to change from the clients, but not to provide them, personally.

Beck and Emery (1985) suggested a procedure called "point-counterpart," which can facilitate the attainment of this goal. The clients in the group, one by one, play roles to try to convince the group therapist, who plays the role of a highly resistant client, to view the problem as one worth working on. Then the group therapist suggests that each person actually draw a balance scale.

Four questions are asked of the clients, who are asked to write down their answers. What are the advantages of not doing anything about one's present situation? What are the disadvantages of changing one's present behavior? What are the advantages of changing the present behavior? And what are the disadvantages of not changing the behavior? The clients in the group then simply list the answers to each of the questions. The clients are encouraged to borrow other clients' ideas that reflect their positions, and add them to their lists. They are asked to give a weight on a scale of 1 to 9 in terms of the importance to them of each item. Then the answers to 1 and 2 are placed on the balance scale on the negative side, and the answers to 3 and 4 are placed on the positive side.

In the process of weighing costs and benefits, different people place different values on a given outcome or a given reward. The clients are advised that the weights attributed to their answers may change over time. The group therapist is careful not to direct or suggest answers. Everyone is encouraged to put on their lists only those answers they believe are accurate for them personally. In the presentation to the group, the clients may suggest additional answers to each other. In this exercise, the reasons for lack of motivation and the seeds for increasing motivation are made explicit.

Eliciting and reinforcing self-motivational statements. Miller and Rollnick (1991) identified four types of self-motivational statement: a problem recognition statement, an expression of concern about the problem, an expression of intention to change, and an optimistic statement about change. Each type suggests increasingly greater motivation for change. The question for the group therapist is how such statements can be evoked in the group.

Miller and Rollnick (1991) suggested a number of strategies that are applicable not only in individual treatment but also in the group: direct questioning, asking clients to elaborate on an issue brought to the group, using extremes, looking back to when times were better, looking forward to a time when the problem might not exist, exploring the incompatibility with personal goals of present behavior, and use of paradoxical statements, such as, "I am not convinced from what you say that you really have a problem."

To teach clients in groups to recognize self-motivational statements, one exercise therapists can use is to create two fictional cases in which the simulated clients are at various levels of motivation and ask the clients in the group to identify the degree of motivation of each individual to change and the evidence for their judgments. Then the clients identify in each case the potential or actual self-motivating statements the clients might make. Finally, the clients compare themselves to the two cases to indicate how they are different. Clients are then encouraged to identify self-motivational statements they have heard people in the group make, without identifying who those persons were.

To reinforce such statements, the group therapist encourages clients to note when an individual client makes one. This serves to reinforce the positive statements of the client and also to model such statements for the others. The group therapist may also point out these statements as he or she hears them. A modified version of the cognitive modeling sequence can be used to encourage self-enhancing motivational statements or to reinforce those statements. This sequence originally consists of setting the scene, cognitive modeling with thought stopping and cognitive rehearsal, group feedback, and fading.

Removing barriers to active client involvement in treatment. If clients can't get to the session, the above techniques cannot be used. Practical barriers such as lack of transportation, need for child care, lack of any small group experience, prohibitive cost of treatment, night sessions in unsafe neighborhoods, and inadequate facilities for the disabled or the elderly may prevent a person from attending the group. With adequate funding, many of these barriers may be overcome. In working with lower socioeconomic groups, it is sometimes also helpful if the group sessions are held in neighborhoods closer to the residences of the clients. Clients with limited education may need additional help in using learning materials dispensed in the group. The role of the group therapist is to identify and deal with these matters before the group begins. Some problems may not be discovered until a person misses a group session. The group can then be asked to help deal with the barriers.

Psychological barriers, such as resistance to the pressure of a peer group to continue the undesirable behavior, a fear of meeting new people, and previous bad experiences in groups are more difficult to deal with. If the prospective client gets to the first session or even a pregroup interview, these issues can be identified and discussed. The therapist responds with empathy rather than problem solving or confrontation. The participants are encouraged to try out a few sessions to determine whether what they feared might not be absent from this particular group. Pointing out differences between this and other types of group or individual therapy may also be supportive. If the barriers are assessed as products of the normal reluctance of many people to new experiences, merely normalizing their ambivalence (see above) may be an adequate response.

To assess the existing barriers, after a brief introduction in which barriers are identified, the therapist asks the clients to present any barriers that prevented them from coming to sessions or restricted their participation in any way in previous treatment groups or individual sessions. They are also asked if they anticipate these or other barriers to participating actively in the given group. The therapist is careful to elicit the opinions of the clients and not to provide them personally. The group therapist may suggest some additional possible barriers. Then strategies are developed together with the client for dealing with the more apparent of these barriers.

Fear of a breach of confidentiality may also be a barrier for some. A discussion of the need for confidentiality of whatever people discuss in the group is also emphasized as a way of reducing this threat. Although confidentiality in groups cannot be guaranteed, the clients are assured that everything will be done to increase the probability that the rule of confidentiality will not be breeched, and their cooperation is enlisted. Group discussion of the problems involved when confidentiality is not maintained should be a topic of early sessions. In many of our groups, a contract is signed by the clients and the group therapist that nothing presented will be discussed outside of the group. The therapist, however, warns that she or he is required by law to report felonious acts to the police.

Ongoing measurement of the level of motivation. One additional strategy for increasing any positive behavior is simply measuring it and responding appropriately to the measurement. We have found that this is also true for motivation. One can observe whether assignments are being completed, whether clients are prepared for sessions, and whether they participate in the session in a positive and constructive way. One can count the number of self-motivational statements made by clients in each session. It is also possible to ask the clients to do this themselves. However, we have found that clients tire quickly of long checklists, so we have devised a two-item checklist to give us an indication of level of motivation in a group (see Figure 2). This two-item checklist and open-ended questions are given at the end of each session. The results provide a basis for discussing motivation at the following session. One method is to ask the clients in the group at the end of each session to ascertain how motivated they are to work on their problem on a 9-point scale. This leaves the definition of motivation or commitment to each person within the parameters contained in the question. To test the reliability of the people's self-measurements, the group therapist should rate each person in the group on the same scale. We have also asked clients to estimate the motivation of the group as a whole. Broad discrepancies between group therapists' and clients' views, and between self-assessment and group assessment of level of motivation, can be discussed with the group as part of the treatment.

Two last measures that can be used to estimate the motivation of clients in the group are the rate of attendance and the dropout rate. The following principles deal directly with that index.

Follow-up contacts. To increase attendance, a telephone call to clients reminds them of the session. Miller and Rollnick (1991) noted that the risk of a client dropping out was highest following the first session in alcohol treatment. This reflects our own experience in all kinds of treatment groups. Miller and Rollnick also reviewed research that clearly demonstrated that a simple personal phone call before the second session and after a client has missed a session dramatically lowered the dropout rate (e.g., Nirenberg, Sobell, & Sobell, 1989). In group counseling for domestic abuse perpetrators, Taft, Murphy, Elliott, and Morrel (2001) also demonstrated that supportive telephone calls and handwritten notes from therapist to client at the outset of treatment and after any missed sessions were associated with a significant reduction in treatment dropout and a significant increase in session attendance. For this reason, these types of intersession contact are highly recommended, and though time consuming, appear to be highly cost effective. In groups, the clients themselves may be enlisted to assist in these tasks between session contacts.

Figure 2. Identifying the level of motivation

1. How committed are you right now to carrying out suggestions or changes recommended in the group? (circle the number closest to your level of commitment to change).

1-----------2----------3----------4----------5----------6----------7----------8----------9

| Not at all | Very little | Somewhat | Quite a bit | Extremely |

2. How committed did you think the group as a whole was at this session to carrying out suggestions or changes recommended in the group? (circle the number closest to the average level of commitment)

1-----------2----------3----------4----------5----------6----------7----------8----------9

| Not at all | Very little | Somewhat | Quite a bit | Extremely |

FIGURE 2 Identifying the Level of Motivation.

SUMMARY

In this article a number of overlapping principles have been pointed out, the application of which appears to enhance the motivation of clients in group treatment. Although developed for the most part by Miller and Rollnick (1991, 2002) for individuals, this article demonstrates how many of these same principles can make use of the group in facilitating their application. To apply these principles in groups, group exercises have been designed to train the clients in the implementation of each of the principles and to provide them practice in implementing them in a safe environment.

In spite of their research support of applying motivational interviewing to individual therapy with patients who abuse alcohol, cigarettes, and other substances (Miller & Rollnick, 2002), to our knowledge there is as yet no systematic research that supports the efficacy of these principles as they are applied in social work with groups. Such research is certainly called for. At present, only clinical experience and extrapolation from research on individuals supports the incorporation of these principles into group work with clients whose motivation seems low.

REFERENCES

Antonuccio, D., Lewinsohn, P., & Breckenridge, J. (1987). Therapist variables related to cohesiveness in a group treatment for depression. *Small Group Behavior*, *18*(4), 557–564.

Beck, A. T., & Emery, G. (1985). *Anxiety disorders and phobias*. New York: Basic Books.

Beckham, E. (1992). Predicting patient dropout in psychotherapy. *Psychotherapy*, 29(2), 177–182.

Bednar, R., Melnick, J., & Kaul, T. (1974). Risk, responsibility, and structure. *Journal of Counseling Psychology*, 21(1), 31–37.

Bernard, H., & Drob, S. (1989). Premature termination. *Group*, 13(1), 11–22.

Bostwick, G. (1987). Where's Mary? *Social Work with Groups*, 10(3), 117–132.

Budney, A. J., Higgins, S. T., Radonovich, K. J., & Novy, P. L. (2000). Adding voucher-based incentives to coping skills during treatment for marijuana dependence. *Journal of Consulting and Clinical Psychology*, 68(6), 1051–1072.

Burke, B. L., Arkowitz, H., & Dunn, C. (2002). The efficacy of motivational interviewing and its adaptations. In R. M. William & S. Rollnick (Eds.), *Motivational interviewing: Preparing people for change* (pp. 217–250). New York: Guilford Press.

Duan, C., & Hill, C. E. (1996). The current state of empathy research. *Journal of Counseling Psychology*, 43(3), 261–274.

Dutton, D. G. (1986). The outcome of court-mandated treatment for wife assault. *Violence and Victims*, 1(3), 163–175.

Edleson, J. L., & Grusznski, R. J. (1989) Treating men who batter. *Journal of Social Service Research*, 12, 3–22.

Liberman, M. A., Yalom, I., & Miles, M. (1973). *Encounter groups*. New York: Basic Books.

Liberman, R. (1970). A behavioral approach to group dynamics. *Behavior Therapy*, 1, 141–175.

Miller, W. R., & Rollnick, S. (1991). *Motivational interviewing: Preparing people to change addictive behavior*. New York: Guilford Press.

Miller, W. R., & Rollnick, S. (2002). *Motivational interviewing: Preparing people for change*. New York: Guilford Press.

Murphy, J., & Cannon, D. (1986). Avoiding early dropouts. *Journal of Psychosocial Nursing*, 24(9), 21–26.

Nirenberg, T. D., Sobell, L. C., & Sobell, M. B. (1989). Effective and inexpensive procedures for decreasing client attrition in an outpatient alcohol treatment program. *American Journal of Drug and Alcohol Abuse*, 7, 73–82.

O'Leary-Kelly, A. M., Martocchio, J. J., & Frink, D. D. (1994). A review of the influence of group goals on group performance. *Academy of Management Journal*, 37(5), 1285–1302.

Rose, S. D. (1998). *Group therapy with troubled youth: A cognitive-behavioral interactive approach*. Thousand Oaks, CA: Sage.

Sethna, E., & Harrington, J. (1971). A study of patients who lapsed from group psychotherapy *British Journal of Psychiatry*, 119, 59–69.

Stewart, L., & Montplaisir, G. (1999). *Reasons for drop-outs among participants in the cognitive skills and anger and other emotions management programs*. Unpublished manuscript.

Taft, C. T., Murphy, C. M., Elliott, J. D., & Morrel, T. M. (2001). Attendance-enhancing procedures in group counseling for domestic abusers. *Journal of Counseling Psychology*, 48(1), 51–60.

Wright, P. M., & Kacmar, K. M. (1994). Goal specificity as a determinant of goal commitment and goal change. *Organizational Behavior and Human Decision Processes, 59*(2), 242–261.

Yalom, I. V. (1985). *The theory and practice of group psychotherapy.* New York: Basic Books.

Zweben, A., & Zuckoff, A. (2002). Motivational interviewing and treatment adherence. In R. M. William & S. Rollnick (Eds.), *Motivational interviewing: Preparing people for change* (pp. 299–332). New York: Guilford Press.

Index

Printed in the United States
by Baker & Taylor Publisher Services